Am I Really Hungry?

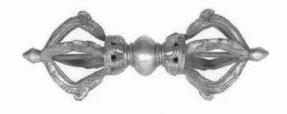

6th Sense Diet
Intuitive Eating

A Fine Tuning Book

Jane Bernard

Am I Really Hungry? 6th Sense Diet : Intuitive Eating

Copyright 2011 by Jane Bernard

Am I Really Hungry? is a psychological and intuitive approach to eating and dieting. Ten tools are provided that keep you aware of your intuition. Learn how to eat when you're hungry and stop when you're not. Eating intuitively is liberating. It frees your mind from trying to control your body and puts you in sync with yourself. It's a freedom, a release and an unburdening that will change your life.

The information contained in this book is intended to be educational and not for diagnosis, prescription, or treatment of any health disorder whatsoever. The information should not replace consultation with a competent healthcare professional. The author and publisher expressly disclaim responsibility for any adverse effects arising from misuse of the information contained in this book.

LLCN- 2011906116

Copyright © 2011 Jane Bernard
All rights reserved.
ISBN-10: 1461098769
ISBN-13: 978-1461098768

DEDICATION

This book is dedicated to every person who has the courage
to be true to their heart.

ACKNOWLEDGMENTS

This book could not have been written without the generous support of my family and friends who I thank with humility and a twinkle of Love.

I am especially grateful to and want to thank the women and men who worked with me and were willing to let go of diet dogma to use the intuitive tools to lose weight.

Sincere appreciation also goes to the many people who contributed their knowledge to the book and to those I interviewed who were open about eating hot buttons and their struggles with dieting. Thank you to the celebrity chefs for the delicious comfort food recipes and to Dr. Judy Kuriansky who suggested this be published. Without these people, I would not have a book.

And importantly, I would like to thank my cousin Linda and my brother Ralph Cohen who have been my heart through this process.

Am I Really Hungry?

6th Sense Diet : Intuitive Eating

Table of Contents

Part 3: Rewards

Am I Really Hungry?
6th Sense Diet : Intuitive Eating

Introduction

"There is no use trying, said Alice;
one can't believe impossible things.
I dare say you haven't had much practice, said the Queen. When I
was your age, I always did it for half an hour a day. Why, sometimes
I've believed as many as six impossible things before breakfast."[1]

Lewis Carroll

Want to quit worrying about calories or lists of forbidden foods? The 6th Sense Diet is liberating. There's no counting calories or lists of forbidden foods, and no inner critic. Instead of calories and rules, you get 10 tools for eating intuitively. Discover solutions for weight problems and begin long-term satisfaction with yourself and your body starting with chapter 1.

Know what you want to eat by listening to your 6th sense. In chapter 14, different types of hunger are explained to help you learn what your body needs is what you want to eat. Intuition is your 6th sense. It's a grounding and arousal sense you can depend on to stay clear about food choices so you feel and look great.

Tired of feeling guilty and frustrated around eating? No more guilt or frustration around eating because in chapter 15, you gain insights into how emotional reactions to eating interfere with real needs, and you will learn to use intuitive tools to put an end to confusion created by old habits.

Want to stop binging, have less bloat and fewer mood swings? Who doesn't want more energy, less bloat, fewer mood swings, to stop binging and think more clearly? In chapter 16 you'll understand how to recognize signals in your life that keep you in control.

Learn how to eat when you're hungry and stop when you're not. You won't be told what to eat, but you will learn to understand when you're hungry and when to stop. In chapter 20, find out how to end the tormenting experience of being obsessed with food. This is the last diet book you'll ever have to buy.

Find new pleasure in eating without the emotional baggage of dieting. By using intuitive tools, your emotional hot buttons around eating, diet and maintaining your healthy weight become a thing of the past. Chapter 22 reveals how to take the pleasure of eating to a whole new level. As you transform into being an intuitive eater, being honest with yourself is the compass that eliminates confusion.

Want to learn some great new comfort food recipes that celebrity chefs cook for themselves? There's a mouth-watering mac and cheese recipe from celebrity chef Kerry Simon and a delicious diet-friendly fruit and nut cobbler from Australian diet guru, Annette Sym. In chapter 27, celebrity chefs from around the world share their comfort food recipes.

Join intuitive eaters everywhere to enjoy meals, lose weight, learn about yourself and use your 6th sense to make the "impossible" possible. No more yo-yo dieting. Connect with your body in a whole new way and get rid of dieting for good!

If you're willing to stop dieting, tune into your body and start trusting your 6th sense, you're on the way to a natural and empowering transformation. I promise that the journey will be satisfying and the reward, a long-term reality.

Part 1: **A New Beginning** is the key to launching your success. Think of the rest of this book as a buffet. Browse the table of contents and pick what feels relevant

- Follow your intuition.

- Question things proactively, not defensively.

- Try things. The idea is to get what your body needs and also what you want.

There is no doubt you will be using your intuition and making a lot of discoveries about how amazing you are.

"50% of what we know is wrong. The problem is that we don't know which 50% it is." Timothy Noakes PhD

Chapter 1: Intuition, Our 6th Sense

When it counts, people use their intuition. Just ask any policeman, doctor, fireman or member of the armed forces. They trust their intuition to know what's really happening. When it comes to intuition, everyone has it. Many people use their 6 senses to stay in touch with their body and stay slim. Our senses are the way of being in direct touch with our body and our world.

As you connect with your intuition it will be like slowly releasing a pressure valve from your eating routine. You'll feel different because you'll look at eating differently. Your attitude towards your body will change.

"Man your ships, and may the force be with you."3 Star Wars, George Lucas

Your 'ships' are the 5 senses: taste, touch, seeing, hearing and smell. The 'force' is your 6th sense: intuition.

The 6th sense is also called intuition, gut feeling, common sense, survival instinct or 'that little voice'. Intuition is an important part of the puzzle of who you are. It is a natural 'GPS', your personal coordinating and guidance system that will get you exactly where you want to be. As you tune into it, you learn about yourself. You realize your brain is not more important to you than your digestive system.

Intuition is a quiet connection with an inner sense of direction that feels like a surge of gentle energy you recognize as being in sync with yourself. You feel grounded. The more you connect, the more rewarding it gets. Like your other 5 senses, intuition is not intellectual; it's instant. This is an inner resource you were born with that is never destructive and only serves your best interests. Intuition is the "force" that connects with and guides what makes eating sense for your best quality of life.

When you "man your ships", you're taking control of your five physical senses by choosing to be completely aware of information you receive from them. This is how to notice what you take for granted. Ultimately, you feel more alert. In the beginning, eating using your eyes, ears, nose, mouth and tongue is literally an eye opener.

Your 6th sense maintains communication between all 5 senses and connects this input to your body, mind and heart. Look at your hand and think of your five fingers as your 5 senses, and your palm as intuition.

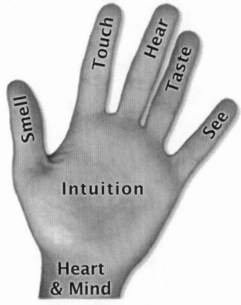

Your fingers work together because of your palm. If you hurt your palm, it's hard to catch a ball or hold a baby. If you ignore your 6th sense, the other 5 senses cannot work to your fullest advantage. This leaves you physically, intellectually and emotionally handicapped.

The palm is a connector and an enabler, and so is the 6th sense. Intuition connects what we sense, communicates this with our mind and body, and makes us aware of opportunities that serve our best interest - all in an instant without thinking.

The 6th sense is an arousal and grounding sense that takes what you experience and pushes it up a notch, making it clearer. It unifies and balances perceptions so you can respond fully to immediate needs. The survival instinct is an obvious time when you use your 6th sense.

The job of all of our senses is to provide immediate pleasure and protection. The senses ground and focus what we do by keeping us connected to the present. Intuition gives pleasure and protection by communicating what you sense. At the same time, intuition keeps your mind clear about your priorities so you can be receptive to messages from your body and heart about what you need. This way, intuition creates an internal balance so you remain clear about long-term perspective and priorities as you make eating choices.

Intuition always responds to:

Your Whole Body:

Including its many systems, organs, regenerating qualities, as well as what holds it together – muscles and skin.

All Emotions:

Which speak to you silently and manipulate you physically; can make you cry, bring tears of laughter to your eyes, or make you overeat.

We often call emotions heart.

Your Brain:

Which is your own internal hard drive, with a record of what's been downloaded.

The brain records experiences so we can use them to keep moving forward instead of reliving bad choices.

Intuition works as an inner coordinating and guidance system you can count on for stability, continuity and quality of life, 24/7. As you connect with your 6th sense, you'll recognize a comforting way of being in sync with yourself that feels like confidence. This feeling is your 6th sense.

4 Big Questions:

How does intuitive eating help me lose weight?

Intuitive eating keeps you connected to your constantly changing physical needs and with what you value. This means you eat more wisely and avoid emotional eating. You see and feel the need to lose weight - or not- when you stay connected with your intuition. People gain weight when they disconnect, by ignoring what they sense from their body or their values.

How does it help me keep off weight I lose?

Intuitive eating focuses on quality of life. You have the best quality of life and feel best about yourself at your healthy weight. Intuitive eaters see every meal as an opportunity to maintain their quality of life.

You will keep weight off by staying clear about what matters to you. Knowing when you're hungry, and eating what makes sense, is eating intuitively. Ignoring or not using your intuition means eating choices you later regret. The secret is to know yourself and use intuitive tools to stay connected with who you are. The intuitive tools strengthen physical and emotional links by connecting and balancing your internal systems with your external responsibilities.

Intuitive eating is not a diet; it's a lifestyle. A quality of life is created and reinforced by using the custom-tailored intuitive tools. You stay where you want to be.

Is it hard?

All change is initially hard. Intuitive eating gets easier as you increasingly recognize, trust and depend on the tools. The effect snowballs. Since intuitive choices mean you feel and look good, it becomes natural. Eating intuitively is a win-win situation.

How can eating intuitively make me aware of portion control or healthy eating?

Because intuition connects with what matters most, you recognize what feels good to your body.

Your mind and senses work with your intuition, so you see and know what portion is comfortable and healthy for your body. Since intuition is a clearinghouse for what you've experienced, as well as what you feel and sense, portion control and eating what your body needs becomes automatic.

Intuitive eating is not rigid. Instead of rules about portion control, there are tools custom-tailored to your constantly changing needs.

A recent headline on BBC News stated *"The diet business: Banking on Failure"* The article continues: *The diet business has never been in better shape- unlike many of its customers. But with research suggesting 95% of the slimmers regain the weight, does the diet industry rely on our failure to make it's profits?1*

Dieters see each meal as a step along the path to a long-term weight loss goal. Intuitive eaters see each meal as an immediate important source of energy and nourishment. Your intuitive long-term goal is a lifestyle of maintaining a comfortable healthy body.

Dieters are often advised to plan meals a week in advance. This is counter-intuitive. It's impossible to know on Monday what your body will want or need for lunch on Wednesday. Intuition, with your 5 senses keeps you in touch with the present, which is where your body is all the time. This is how you know when you're hungry and what you want to eat.

The word 'diet' originated in the 14th century to describe the restricted intake of prisoners. *"They were fed a diet of bread and water."* This is the 21st century. Today, every species except us eats intuitively.

Note: We're the only ones who diet, and we're unhealthy because of our eating habits. It's time to eat intuitively.

Intuitive eaters don't force themselves to eat what their body and senses reject. According to the New York Times, if you force yourself to eat something boring or unappetizing, your body absorbs up to 70% <u>less</u> nutrition.5 So don't do that to yourself. It's healthy to enjoy what you eat.

Whether you realize it or not, intuition is always present coordinating everything in your life as it happens. Everyone, at least once, suddenly has intuitively jumped out of harm's way.

A study done by the Army Research Institute confirms that in a dangerous situation, intuition sends out an alarm so you react physically before understanding in your mind, recognizing why. (Dr. Jennifer Murphy, IED Study, Army Research Institute, 2009)[6] This means you can trust your intuition. You can count on it as a clearinghouse where eating options crystallize and priorities are realized. Using the 6th sense, you make eating choices to keep on track. That's empowering. The Catch 22 is: most of us barely notice our intuition.

Inner Voice & Inner Dialogue

Your inner voice is not the same as your inner dialogue. Your inner voice is your 6th sense. It doesn't pass judgments or make you feel bad. Your inner voice guides and protects your best interests without manipulating your emotions. Inner dialogue manipulates your emotions.

In the beginning, it's natural to confuse inner voice with inner dialogue. However, as you learn to use the intuitive tools, you will easily recognize the differences and will discover it's natural and more comfortable to stay clearly in tune with your inner voice. It's intuitive to really know yourself and recognize what's right for you.

Inner voice:

- Intuition is your inner voice. It's always protective. You can tap into it any time to connect with feelings of self-control around eating. It's both gentle and persistent at the same time. Sometimes it feels like common sense. Sometimes it just feels more relaxing. With practice, you can easily recognize and depend on it. Once you believe from experience that your intuition is the winning ticket, you'll hold on to it tighter.

Inner Dialogue:

- Inner dialogue is what you have heard from outside yourself, repeated inside your head. It is what you hear on the news, what your mother said, what you were told by the doctor, what you read and what you've been taught going through the School of Life.

- Inner dialogue is usually emotionally driven. It can be destructive, restrictive or demeaning. It is the voices of others who we either respect or fear. These voices are teachers and each comes from their unique perspective, but not yours!

- Often inner dialogue doesn't feel intuitively 'right'. Always choose your inner voice.

There's an expression: You can never judge a person until you've walked in their shoes. This also applies to judging yourself: Don't pre-judge yourself by what others think or say. Walk your own walk in your shoes.

Connect with Your Body

Thinking about eating strictly in terms of calories and rigid diets keeps you focused in your head and misses the point of connecting with your body when you eat.

*"If you can't solve a problem,
it's because you're playing by the rules." P. Arden*[7]

The fact is nobody rules your hunger or your body but you. Intuitively, every meal is personal and custom-tailored by you for your needs. Trusting your inner voice frees you from rules imposed by the experience of others, so you can create ways of eating based on your life realities. For example, you may be most hungry when you wake up and would prefer a light dinner, or you may not feel the need for lunch.

Your body will tell you when you're hungry. Your inner voice also frees you to adopt rules others have discovered that intuitively feel right for you. As you learn to recognize the difference between your inner voice and inner dialogue, you get a refreshed perspective on how to eat.

Use your 5 senses when you wake up to notice how you're feeling. Start with breakfast that makes sense for your lifestyle and physical needs. Shake up your eating routine and notice what's going on. Does your food please you? Or do you feel nothing except that it's functional and you need to eat?

What to do:

- If you feel nothing, then no matter what the size of the portion, cut it in half and place ½ on another plate. Then, put that away, or if you're eating out, ask for a doggie bag. Think about options that might be more appealing.

- If you feel pleased, enjoy eating your meal. Remember, enjoying your food enhances the digestive process, so you get more nutritional value when you eat.

- Use curiosity with your senses to recognize and feel the benefits of what you eat or drink. Visualize yourself with your ideal body in your ideal environment, and then feed your ideal body.

- Think about how you are treating yourself with dignity by respecting your body. You'll feel good.

Decide to recognize what you notice through your senses. Start with your sense of smell. Before food enters your mouth, use patience to pause to smell it. Since you don't put food in your mouth without smelling it, you are eating at a slower healthier pace. The result is you will eat less.

As you use your nose to recognize a smell, it's automatic to look at what you smell. Then, what you see is recognized in your brain, which is where you draw a conclusion about it and use common sense about eating it.

For example: a tray of muffins is passed to you at a breakfast meeting. You automatically pick one up and bring it towards your mouth. Now, hold it there and sniff. Recognize a sweet fruity smell. Hmnnn. Look and see it's a blueberry muffin. Notice it's bigger than your fist. You think, I like this muffin, but it's really big and sweet. Using your intuitive tools to connect, you decide you like your body better than the muffin. But, the muffin smells and looks delicious, so you use prudence along with determination to cut it in half, twice, and slowly enjoy the smell, sight and taste of one of the pieces. You know what you're eating and you know why you're eating it. You're enjoying it, and won't have regrets.

Exercises to be an intuitive eater:
- Take time to recognize all 5 physical senses when you're around food.

- Hear what makes sense. When it's time to eat, listen to your body, heart and mind. Listen to your whole self without prejudice. You know what's really in your best interests.

- Smell food before putting it in your mouth. Does it smell inviting? Greasy? Fresh? Bad? Be curious. Learn about what you're eating by smelling it. If the food doesn't smell right, it isn't. Let your nose protect you and help to guide your choices.

- Taste food as you chew it. The digestive process starts in your mouth. Chewing food burns calories. Also, you taste more when you chew with your mouth closed. And, as you taste your food, enjoy it. Be thankful for it.

- It's intuitive to think about what food is giving you: energy, strength, health, nourishment and pleasure. In fact, it takes 15 minutes before your brain gets the message from your stomach that you've eaten. Use patience. Take your time and you will eat less.

- Pause to visualize your ideal healthy body. Imagine what it feels like to be fit: how easy to move, how much energy you ideally have during the day. Visualize yourself with your ideal body in the morning before you get out of bed. How do you look? How do you feel?

- Other good times to visualize your ideal body are when you're taking a shower, about to go to sleep, or if you're bored. You will discover that the more detail you imagine, the easier it is to connect with your ideal body. Just imagine having your ideal body in your ideal environment for a few seconds; the image will stay with you.

- Visualize and feed your ideal healthy body when you eat and you'll discover the freedom and desire to make new eating choices.

Use your senses to develop your taste in a way that feels right and makes sense for your lifestyle and eating goals. Try:

- Instead of eating candy, have a sliced apple; it probably costs less than the candy bar and will fill you up longer.

- Instead of French fries, eat a baked potato.

- If you crave carbs but want to lose weight and have plateaued, break the roll at dinner in half, then break it in half again and slowly eat a quarter of it instead of the whole thing. Have the remainder of it removed from the table.

- It's common to mistake thirst for hunger. Instead of eating in the middle of the night, drink half a glass of water – even if you don't think you're thirsty. Water is healthy. Your body uses it to flush out impurities and there are no calories.

- Juice has as many calories as soda, so limit intake to 8oz. a day. Try diluting juice with water; it will last longer and you will benefit from drinking more water and less sugar.

- If you tend to eat fast and to eat big portions, try to drink a full glass of water before each meal. This will slow you down.

The emotional relationship with food is very personal. Emotionally you may justify eating a piece of cake at midnight because you "deserve it". What you deserve is to feel loved. Putting food in your body that will distort your appearance or make your stomach hurt is not an act of love. In fact, it's perverted hostility. Use your mind to connect with your body to get a clear picture. Use tenacity and courage to be kind to yourself.

What you see, hear, taste, feel and smell as you eat connects with what you know and feel about yourself. Intuitively, you want to look good and feel healthy. Focus is the magnifying lens in your intuitive tool chest. It highlights your eating concerns and priorities. Using focus burns calories.

So why is it so hard to be my ideal weight? It's hard because of confusion. Confusion occurs when there's a disconnect from your intuition.

Why eat a portion that is twice as large as I need? When you only focus on calories, you are not staying in touch with yourself physically. Being disconnected from your body is counter-intuitive.

Why eat when I'm not hungry? You have habits that are socially and commercially ingrained that ignore your heart, mind and body.

Why eat what isn't good for my body? You don't know what to eat. Soon you will recognize what is good for you. When you stay in touch with your body, you can try different 'dieting' suggestions to see what works for you.

Using intuition makes it easier to cope with life's surprises. When it comes to meals, we're often faced with the unexpected. Connecting with your 6th sense means comfortably making healthy choices.

More Facts about Intuition:

Animals eat instinctively without thinking about what or how much. People are able to relate to eating differently than animals because intuition works with our conscious mind. You can think when you eat. Use curiosity and prudence to connect with and benefit from your past experience.

Wanting to connect with intuitive eating is the beginning of unlocking old habits that no longer serve you. The key to connecting is self-respect. Self-respect means that you're honest with yourself. It takes a commitment to yourself.

"Unless you believe, you will not understand."[8] St. Augustine

You don't just believe with your mind; you also believe with your heart. That's why a person can 'convince you' about something, but it still won't 'feel right'. That feeling is your inner voice. Experience shows that when you fully believe in yourself, you can depend on finding strength that is beyond your 5 senses.

Really believing is cellular, which means it runs through your whole self. It's powerful because believing keeps us open to success. Tuning in to your intuition is tuning in to your natural power base. Results are tangible. With practice and believing, intuitive eating becomes automatic.

Your Conscience:

Our inner voice has been called the conscience. The writer Henry Fielding said, our conscience is the only incorruptible thing about us.[9] Intuition is not corruptible. It is a consistent personal beacon of your exclusive truth.

As you use intuitive tools, fine tune your senses and commit to trusting your 6th sense, you ultimately trust yourself. This is a bold kind of self-love. Try it.

"What we need is to use what we have."[10] *Susan Sontag*

Use your brain, but don't let it bully your intuition:

When our brain rules, the tendency is to find comfort in habits. It's like being on auto-drive and we've all been there. You can either learn from the past or repeat it. It's easy to get into mind-driven eating habits. You "think" you're comfortable, but you're not.

Remember the story of the man who felt so good after he stopped banging his head against the wall? Before that, he felt just the same as always.

Balancing Act

Intuitive eating is a balancing act. It's natural to balance thoughts with feelings in order to maintain priorities for eating choices that work for your body. Because intuition connects the senses, mind and heart, a perfect system is created. You experience this as feeling alert. That feeling is your intuition.

Common sense is the meeting place where past experience and what you are currently sensing comes together and your best interests are served. Common sense feels good because it keeps you in touch with what's real. You'll discover that intuitive eating feels like 'common sense'.

Last night, I had a lobster roll dinner with a close friend who is a chronic yo-yo dieter. Without pausing as he finished, my friend ordered a second. Thirty minutes later, while the evening was still young, he was uncomfortable. His digestive system was thrown out of balance by his gorge and it surely put a damper on our evening.

If he used foresight and dignity, my friend would not have had 2 lobster rolls. Instead, he would have savored the delicious experience of one and then been able to enjoy the rest of the evening.

We are duped into believing that more is better and that more is the same as more satisfying. Not true.

Balance is the key to satisfaction.

- Tenacity is the intuitive way to make a commitment that gives us the chance to succeed. Self-doubt is a form of self-sabotage. There is a fact about human nature which is: until we believe we are doing the right thing, there is the chance we will draw back. Don't take that chance. Make a commitment to be true to yourself by staying alert.

- Use your senses to pay attention to what you notice. Remember, you may ignore facts, but you can't change them.

- Media targets senses and emotions with glamorous, slim, smiling people eating huge stacks of pancakes or drinking thick, calorie-intensive cool drinks. The whole point of these commercials is to make you want to eat and drink.

- Commercials plant seeds of desire and doubt by implying that we will be more socially attractive and happier if we follow their example. Language bombards us with: "now". Do it now, enjoy it now, etc. They are selling instant gratification by overeating! That's warped thinking. It's simply not real.

There is an expression that says, if it sounds too good to be true, it is too good to be true. Instant gratification by overeating is an example of this. Part of knowing yourself is recognizing how your senses are being manipulated. Connecting with dignity, determination and courage helps you know yourself.

Everyday pressures dictate our priorities. In the mess of stress, it's often hard to know what to eat. This is when to use patience and pause to use intuitive tools. The pause balances by connecting you with body and mind. Intuitive eating is realizing that what you need is what you really want.

Eating meals without reflecting on options is like filling the tank of a car without looking at the pump. If you put diesel in a gas engine, it clogs up fuel lines and fouls the engine. Eating foods that aren't what your body needs has equally disastrous results. Wrong choices ultimately take up time and lead where you don't want to go. Rushing to eat without reflection means making wrong choices.

Remember when Pepsi ads had the tag line: "It's the pause that refreshes." In everything you do, it's the pause that gives you space to make the right choice.

Connect with your 6th sense and pause to refresh your life. When you eat and reflect about what is really important, energy travels from your heart to your mind. This refreshes your commitment to be clear about what you want.

Intuitive eating is effective, not abusive. It's not about the food, it's about you. It is a kind of self-respect. It's knowing yourself and eating differently. All intuitive eaters maintain their 6th sense connection by depending on intuitive tools to overcome eating challenges.

Factoid:

Dr. Alan Hirsch, neurologist, psychiatrist and Neurological Director of the Smell and Taste Treatment and Research Foundation in Chicago, has done studies on taste and weight loss that reveal the effect taste and smell have on the amount of food we eat. Dr. Hirsch discovered a trend where patients who had lost their sense of smell often gained 10 to 30 pounds.[12] As a result he theorized that if loss of smell leads to weight gain, the opposite might also be true - that enhancing smell can promote weight loss. And it does.

Your nose knows. As you inhale aromas of foods you're being served, remember to connect your anticipation of satisfaction with the sweet smell of diet success.

Chapter 2 : **Intuitive Tools**

"Any sufficiently advanced technology is indistinguishable from magic." Arthur C. Clarke

Intuitive tools effortlessly support your goals for ultimate quality of life. They are a complete system 24/7 and the direct connect with what you want, need and desire. The tools are convenient, useful, save time and money and your body loves them. Does it sound like magic? Start using the tools and feel the magic.

The ten tools are easy to use because you already have them. They work with your body, mind and emotions to keep priorities clear about body goals and eating. Using them connects with the intuitive pleasure of being in control when you eat. Achieving and maintaining a healthy weight has never been easier.

Doing research for this book, I questioned people struggling with the ups and downs of losing weight and talked to people who don't diet but were generally slim, to learn why people eat. The answers were surprising. Instead of learning about what to eat or how to keep weight off, I learned that eating is intensely personal.

One question I asked was: When you look at a menu how do you choose what to order? Every dieter ordered for taste which worked for me since I was writing about the senses, but my intuition kept nudging me. Even though I related emotionally with the idea of going for taste, there was a bad feeling in my gut making me edgy. Finally, I had an "aha" moment while talking to my girlfriend about a guy she was seeing. She said that he had charisma, money and a sense of humor, but he turned out to be a lying, cheating cad. She looked me right in the eye and said "You can't judge a book by the cover." Zing!

I finally 'heard' my intuition. The taste of food is like the cover of a book. You can't judge a book by the cover and taste often misleads about the goodness of food. As this thought steamrolled through my mind, I realized the relationship with food is like another personal relationship in my life - dating.

Before connecting with my intuition, I was emotionally driven in relationships. I've had amazing hot chemistry only to be dumped, and I've spent an evening being charmed, wined and dined only to find out the guy was married. In my search for the "one" I've learned to get past great chemistry, beautiful eyes and the flash of cash to reach the soul of who I'm seeing, or else I pay. The price is low self-esteem, frustration and a feeling of missed opportunity.

Entering a relationship with food, driven overwhelmingly by taste, is this same sort of a trap. If you know you aren't going to feel good afterwards, there has to be something that will prevent you from going there. Since seeing through a meal's superficial lure of taste, smell and appearance is necessary to get to the soul of intuitive eating, I kept asking questions.

Surprises

People who don't diet and are a healthy weight share two revealing and surprising traits. First, they eat intuitively. They consciously use their senses and connect with their body at mealtime. Second, they count on tools to make and keep food choices in sync with their body goals. They don't think about details of meals in advance. If they feel a need for carbs, they eat carbs. If they feel a need to lose weight, they cut back on portion size and modify eating to achieve short-term body issue goals. The tools make it natural.

It turns out that achieving and maintaining a healthy weight has never been easier. Because intuitive tools work with your body, mind and emotions, the whole picture of eating goals stays clear, and the satisfaction of being in control snowballs. Using the tools with your 5 senses keeps the 6th sense connection open, making choices that protect and give automatic pleasure.

Intuitive eaters eat to live instead of living to eat. They eat what they want when they're hungry. This sounds enviable to a dieter but, in fact, is easier than a diet because it's natural. Intuitive eating sounds glamorous but anybody can do it.

Everyday experience challenges you to prove yourself to yourself and not necessarily in conventional ways. Feelings of confidence, dignity, legitimacy and self-esteem are issues that connect with values and eating. Despite the fact that these feelings are deeply personal, until we connect with our intuition, it's common to be barely aware of them.

Intuition is a total support system and guide that connects with what you value to balance your emotions, appetite and personality. Values are qualities you consider worthwhile for your quality of life. They guide how you think and behave.

"How different our lives are when we really know what is deeply important to us, and, keeping that picture in mind, we manage ourselves each day to be and to know what really matters most."[1]
Stephen Covey

Instead of having rules to follow, intuitive eaters use the tools to be clear about what to eat. They decide feeling good is worth the effort and use their senses to relate to hunger and how their body responds to foods. Intuitive eaters approach each meal guided by a flexible attitude about choice, based on physical hunger.

The artist, Paul Gauguin wrote, *"I shut my eyes in order to see."*[11] If we only use our eyes when we eat, what are we tasting? Use your 5 senses with patience and determination to tune into your body when you eat.

The 10 tools connect with your intuition and values to create the quality of life you want. They work together and with practice, become automatic. You're reconnecting with skills you were born with.

Tool Summary:

Curiosity is being aware. This means having an interest in what you're eating and a flexible attitude about your body's needs. Curiosity is how to stay in control.

Prudence is balancing eating options to guide you to choices that enhance your life. Prudence works with curiosity to show options.

Tenacity is inner drive of resolve - a commitment to be true to yourself, focused on your goals. Tenacity is intuitive muscle power.

Dignity is an attitude of self-respect and self-mastery that is seen in your actions. Dignity maintains your priorities.

Determination is energy experienced as inner drive to follow your intuition. Determination is 'tough love' that powers through stressful eating situations and it's backed by tenacity.

Patience is a stress buster you can count on to gain a clear perspective around food. Patience gives breathing room, and is a respectful way of acknowledging your efforts. It's a form of self-compassion that brings balance.

Foresight is staying connected with the present and also a way of self-control. It's intuitive self-defense.

Self-Discipline is self-reliant and protective. Self-discipline provides stability and self-esteem. Intuitive eaters use this tool as a guide to overcome disappointment.

Courage is the sticking place. It is your lifeline. Courage evaporates fear and overrides doubts. You can tap into it anytime.

The Mystery Tool is an invisible tape that holds together your intuitive perspective and always shines on your total potential.

These tools are your way of connecting and staying connected with your intuition to be a healthy weight. They are lifestyle assets that make eating choices natural, satisfying and rewarding. With practice, they become automatic and you become an intuitive eater.

Every person is born with the gem of intuition. Each intuitive tool is a facet of the gem. Polish your tools and let your intuition sparkle. Once you connect with these, rewarding food choices become obvious and eating stops being stressful. Intuitively there is nothing you can't do.

"Anything is possible if you've got enough nerve."[1] *JK Rowlings*

Chapter 3 : **Curiosity**

Curiosity: Curiosity helps you stay clear about what you want.

Ask the tough questions.

- What makes me feel good?
- When am I afraid?
- Who do I trust?

Physically what do you want?

- To be the biggest "loser"
- To be your optimum physical weight
- To be healthy
- To be prepared for a sport
- To feel great
- To feel fit
- To beat illness
- To change your life
- To ENJOY what you have in your life

As you use curiosity to stay in touch with your body and heart, it re-activates intuitive connections. Discoveries snowball and you'll be amazed at your natural insights.

Intuitive eating goals are taste and quality. Curiosity brings out questions about quality. It has led me to skip low fat brands since I discovered they are often pumped up with less nutritional fillers. I've also learned the tastiest, least expensive produce is whatever is in season and these fresh foods have the most nutritional benefit.

Curiosity is a flexible, open attitude and skill we have as children that fades from disuse. Fine-tuning your 5 senses sharpens it. This power tool for staying in control of eating is like having x-ray vision and super hearing, because curiosity is looking closer and hearing more.

Being aware, is a gentle way of being curious. Use your senses to notice the way your food smells, looks and tastes. When you're aware, you are in control. Questioning is a way of maintaining control. Use curiosity to decide what you really want and what will put you at a disadvantage. Intuitively, you want the advantage and therefore eat to feel good. Curiosity helps you notice what feels good.

Food choices based on using curiosity are spontaneous. Meals aren't decided in advance because intuitive eating is flexible. For dieters, using the tool of curiosity is a big change that takes practice.

Classic 20th century diets dictate what, when and how much to eat. It's a one-size-fits-all reality. Listening to your body or questioning choices is not an option. The result is: dieters are programmed not to be curious and made to believe they do not have self-control around food. When you turn your eating over to a diet plan, you give up responsibility for yourself. Personal power is stripped. Being curious takes it back.

Use curiosity to check in with how you feel before you eat and to recognize what your appetite is telling you. You want a meal that feels good, physically and emotionally, an hour later. Curiosity leads to an adventure with your senses and guides you to make the choice in your best interest. Ultimately, you make the choice that feels right.

Reading labels is smart/curious shopping. Content ingredients are listed by highest amount first. When sugar is the first ingredient, I avoid that food. If I want sugar, I want to know I'm eating it, not have it slipped into food to tease my sense of taste. Shopping for quality includes trying to avoid sodium, saturated and hydrogenated fats and nitrates (a preservative). I avoid food with anything in it that I can't pronounce.

Here are some helpful sites:

goodhousekeeping.com has a section called "Nutrition" which tells how to de-code labels. They also have a section called "Tips", which has helpful short-time videos and my favorite, "Cravings

911", which gave me a recipe called "Quick Chips" as an alternative to my fave deli-style potato chips.

Another way to shop smart is **foodnews.org**. It gives a shoppers' guide to which foods contain pesticides. It isn't necessary to buy only organic to get the best for your body.

Use curiosity to:

Learn about food. For example: Fiber fills you up. A medium sized apple is about 65 calories. A study found people who ate one apple before every meal lost 40% more than those who didn't. Apples have natural sugar as well as fiber, so they give an energy boost and take the edge off hunger. Be curious about buying food. Learn to shop smart.

Practical hints:

- Walking down the aisles of the supermarket when hungry is always a big mistake because everything looks good and it's easy to impulse buy; so have a snack beforehand.

- Make a list of what you need and stick to it.

- Avoid cookie and soda aisles because if these sweets are not in your house, you won't eat them.

- Generally, everything in the produce section is healthy; this is a smart and safe place to start.

Factoids:

- When you cut a carrot it looks like the human eye with the pupil in the middle. Carrots enhance blood flow to the eyes which can improve eye function.

- The tomato has 4 chambers and is red, just like the heart. Tomatoes nurture your heart and blood.

- Grapes hang in clusters that often are the shape of the heart and each grape looks like a cell. Grapes are a profound heart and blood revitalizing food.

- The walnut looks like a little brain with its wrinkles, folds and matching left and right sides. Walnuts help develop more than 3 dozen neuron-transmitters in your brain.

- Kidney beans, which look like human kidneys, help heal and maintain your kidneys.

- Celery, bok choy and rhubarb look like bones and fortify bone strength. Your bones are 23% sodium and so are these foods.

- Eggplant, avocado and pears look like the womb and cervix. They also help fortify womb and cervix health. Interesting fact: It takes exactly 9 months for an avocado to go from blossom to ripened fruit.

- Figs, which are full of seeds, hang in pairs when they grow. These fruits are reported to increase the motion of sperm.

- Sweet potatoes look like your pancreas. The pancreas is where our body makes insulin and other digestive hormones and sweet potatoes are considered tops in nutrition. They are a low glycemic food which means good for diabetics and for controlling blood sugar.

- Grapefruits, oranges, most citrus fruits look like mammary glands. Eating these helps the movement of fluid from lymph glands in and out of the breasts.

Chapter 4: **Prudence**

Prudence is eating by comparing options based on what you want from your meal for your body. It keeps you feeling balanced by showing that you have options. You always have a choice. When you feel balanced, you feel control.

Prudence is used for comparison-shopping. You go shopping with a friend but don't buy the same jeans because you have different bodies and different needs. When you buy new jeans, you compare styles, colors and prices. You look at what's available and try on several to see what looks good and lets you feel your best. The same is true of eating options- what might work for your friend, might not look good on you.

Use prudence to get what you need from what you eat. When you need energy, choose a fortifying meal or if it's time to celebrate, enjoy food you associate with the taste of good times. Options change with circumstances.

Intuitively, prudence and curiosity work together. When it comes to eating, size matters. You can choose how much to eat by looking at it. If it's bigger than your fist, it's a prudent choice not to eat the whole thing.

If you have high cholesterol and choose to avoid foods with cholesterol, it's prudent. When an intuitive eater who is watching his weight, chooses to have a potato with dinner as a carb and decides not to eat the delicious roll offered at the same time, he's using the tool of prudence. Using prudence guides you to make choices that 'feel' right.

Prudent: acting with or showing care and thought for the future

When you're accustomed to being told what to eat and how much to eat, at first, using intuitive prudence is not easy or natural. However, ultimately, it is easier to listen to your body than to fight it.

It's healthier to tune in to your needs than to ignore them. One reason intuitive eating works is because it's custom-tailored to your body. In these busy times, it really helps to pause (patience) and use prudence to reconnect with your intuitive self. Good news is that instead of this being time-consuming, it ultimately saves time. When you make balanced choices, you don't make mistakes. Mistakes are time-consuming. By pausing before you eat to use curiosity and prudence while you choose your food, you reinforce your sense of self-worth. This is a direct intuitive eating connection. It's power.

A Disconnect

Classic dieting takes control of eating by removing choices. The result is you put food into your body without relating to your hunger. This is a disconnect from your body. Unfortunately, when you disconnect from your body, you abuse it.

An eating disconnect occurs when the focus is on the emotional connection with food. Emotion-driven eating ignores physical and personal needs. It's often a knee-jerk reaction to events in life, which may have nothing to do with your physical hunger. Prudence is its foil. Using prudence keeps you aware of options and helps stop emotional urges from sabotaging eating choices.

Eating pushes expected and unexpected emotional buttons. Prudence puts you in charge of those buttons.

Excess is never prudent since it's the opposite of balance. Still, excess happens. It's part of learning and growing. Observe it with curiosity - and not with criticism - and learn. Forgive excess and note unpleasant side effects. Learning from mistakes means you don't repeat them. If you make a food choice that feels bad, it is bad.

Taking control of yourself feels good. Choose to celebrate your body by eating for energy and strength. You will enjoy it. Go for the energy boost of prudence. It will save many regrets in the long run. It will also give some delicious surprises.

Prudence directly impacts you:

- Financially- While food shopping or eating, prudent choices help put more money in your pocket and less calories in your stomach. The tool of prudence helps you use knowledge you gain from being curious to make eating choices that feel good to your wallet and your body.

- Time management - Often time management issues are the result of tunnel vision or selective hearing. Prudence connects with your body, mind, heart and senses so you are aware of options. There is always enough time to make choices that make you feel good when you choose what you are going to eat, and take the time to eat into consideration, to eat food that will give you energy for the lifestyle you want.

- Variety of menu alternatives - Since prudence connects with curiosity, you try new things and these create new connections with your body, because eating is ultimately a physical experience. Prudence shows two options: one familiar, and one 'good for us' that supposedly is also tasty, and curiosity says, why not try it? New experiences stimulate your mind and your stomach. Plus, you are much more apt to taste and smell food that is unfamiliar. You will grow by being prudent and in the process, learn that limits are for the limited.

Use prudence to:

- Practice portion control by considering alternatives. My friend asks for a second plate when served a huge slice of cake or even a huge main course. She puts the portion that makes sense for her on the second plate and asks to have the remainder removed from the table. She doesn't take home 'doggie bags' because she doesn't want to have temptation in her refrigerator. When you think about it, it becomes obvious that there is more than one way to do just about anything.

- Judge the quality of foods you buy and the quality of foods you eat. Use your senses to make prudent decisions by staying aware of what foods satisfy your body and what foods don't feel right. Prudence helps avoid the trap of forming unconscious eating habits.

- Balance eating choices by letting your best interests become apparent. For example, at a buffet it's a wise choice to first focus on protein like roast beef, grilled or baked fish, chicken or lamb dishes. Next choose your vegetables, but avoid potato, pasta and three-bean salads while trying to lose weight.

Factoids:

- Refined, processed and artificially flavored foods are very high in calories. They often are treated with chemicals that confuse feelings of hunger, making it easy to overeat. The chemicals manipulate you to physically feel you want to eat and contribute to obesity. Choose what you eat carefully.

- Your body has a natural ability to balance what you eat with what you need. When you think you're hungry for a snack, instead of having cookies, eat an apple. Slicing it first makes nicer and slower eating. If you're still hungry, eat another apple. **You** decide when you're done. You will know when you have had enough. It's guaranteed you will eat fewer apples than cookies. You can also try this with grapes, carrots or even boiled potatoes. You will discover, using the tools of prudence and curiosity, that you can learn what satisfies you, and you can control your intake.

- Your body uses more energy to digest protein than fat or carbs. That means protein burns more calories. Also, protein energy lasts longer so you don't get hungry as often. Use prudence with curiosity to choose what works best for you.

FirstOurselves.com is a website that says the way to change your relationship with food is to change your relationship with yourself. Karly Randolf Pitman, the founder of FirstOurselves.com, was addicted to sugar, overweight and out of touch with her body before she became an intuitive eater.

Once Karly stopped reading diet books and started listening to her body, she discovered that her intuitive eating choices were unconventional. But, she trusted and listened to her 6th sense and chose foods to eat that she felt her body needed. Now, by eating intuitively, Karly maintains an attractive and healthy weight and continues to feel good about herself. Her very supportive site posts forums for healing binging, body image disorder, and overcoming sugar addiction.

Everyone has a unique body and unique chemistry. This means that what may be the perfect diet for your best friend, may cause you to gain weight. That's why it's important to tune in to food that feels right for you. Eating decisions are personal. Prudence is the tool that works with your experience and physical reality to make your personal best choice

Am I Really Hungry?

Chapter 5 : **Tenacity**

Tenacity is a commitment you make to yourself and until it becomes habit, tenacity requires regular re-booting. It's an "intuitive muscle" and challenges are a form of building strength, like working out. Like all the intuitive tools, this ultimately becomes natural.

Use tenacity to connect directly with your ideal healthy body image. That's the body you'll feed. Imagine how much energy you will have because you make prudent choices, and you'll feel confident. Tenacity works with this vision. It works with your dreams.

Tenacity is the intuitive tool of commitment and resolve to be true to yourself. Lance Armstrong is tenacious. His commitment to an image of being the best he can be is clearly seen by his drive to succeed. Tenacity means: you follow through regardless of odds or external pressures.

A baby learning to walk falls down again, again and again. Because the baby has tenacity, he gets up and tries again, again and again until he walks without falling, and then he can run and climb and move ahead in life. There is a Lance Armstrong and a baby in each of us who can be bold, be brave and work toward our goals.

Tenacity connects with your protective intuitive boundaries. It's a purposefulness that keeps you following through with wise decisions. When you're at a party and there are trays of brownies and bowls of cookies on the table, tenacity helps you choose to stay on the other side of the room. Prudence allows you to eat a brownie if you really want it.

Being tenacious builds:

- Inner strength by reinforcing your natural intuitive connection

- Strength of character by helping you to stay true to yourself

One thing that can never be taken from you is the ability to choose your attitude. Tenacity is an attitude of being true to yourself. With eating, it's not the hand you're dealt, but how you play the game. Tenacity is a lucky charm - only having it has nothing to do with luck. Tenacity is a choice. To practice intuitive eating, make an inner pact to honor yourself.

For example: A fabulous and oversized piece of chocolate mousse cake is placed in front of you. The emotional knee-jerk reaction is to eat it. But tenacity reminds you of how you see yourself and connects with confidence in that image. Use curiosity and look at the cake, smell the chocolate and sugar and feel your juices anticipating it. Then use prudence to see options and make a choice.

You can have none, eat 1/3 of it, take a bite or eat the whole thing. Like Lance Armstrong, you are committed to your image. Like a baby, you have fallen down and are getting up again. How much cake is eaten? Thanks to flexibility and having an open mind because circumstances vary, it's different every time.

Tenacity drives you to keep trying, to keep going. It empowers your dreams by keeping you focused on achieving them. The intuitive dream is to look great, feel good, enjoy eating and enjoy life.

No one gets ahead who quits when it gets tough.

Being tenacious:

- Spurs enthusiasm – because you follow though with the commitment to yourself. When you are running late and need to grab a quick bite, tenacity helps you choose for energy instead of taste.

- Fuels passion – Nothing builds success like success. Tenacity shows you can do what you believe in, when you trust and believe in yourself. This creates momentum, which is exciting.

- Self empowers – Tenacity is staying connected with a singular focus. It connects with intuition to maintain an awareness of purpose and confidence. That's power.

- Sets examples for yourself and others – Be committed to your sense of well-being and the results will excite you and inspire others to follow your example. You may discover that friends, your significant other and even children will "get" your tenacity and join in.

There's something exciting, admirable and inspiring about a person who's committed to doing what feels right. When your choice inspires others to join in, you all can share that huge piece of chocolate cake at the end of the meal.

There are always obstacles in life. It's been said: Fate is something that happens to us and Destiny is how we respond. Honoring yourself includes being realistic about obstacles. Finding an obstacle in the form of a huge slice of birthday cake topped with ice cream is when it's time to connect with what matters.

Let tenacity give you the strength to connect with the way you want your body to appear, and you won't regret not eating the birthday cake. It's not always easy to be the best you can be. But you only get rewarded after you refuse to give up.

Factoid:

- Olives are a low carb fruit. They are credited with reducing symptoms of Lyme disease and Chronic Fatigue Syndrome, are very low calorie (an extra large has 7), contain heart-healthy monounsaturated fats, essential fatty acids and natural anti-oxidants. Eating 3-6 at a time is a nutritious snack.

- Olives were once considered sacred. Over 30,000 visitors a year visit the Olive Tree Museum in Italy. **http://www.museodellolivo.com/eng/index.htm**

Am I Really Hungry?

Chapter 6: **Dignity**

"Sometimes your joy is the source of your smile and sometimes your smile is the source of your joy."[1] Thich Nhat Hanh

Dignity is an attitude of self-respect. It is a tool that works with curiosity to maintain eating priorities. Dignity is not flashy but it is very powerful. It is not found in what you do, but in how you do it. Angelina Jolie, as a mother, has dignity; the 'octuplet mom' does not.

Food keeps coming at a party. An intuitive eater uses tools to cope with the social pressure to eat, drink and be merry. She uses curiosity to check out the food and balances her emotional response by pausing to reflect on physical hunger and nourishment goals before considering her choices. This is how she maintains an attitude of dignity.

Before going to the party she eats a protein snack so she won't feel 'starved'. This prudent choice protects herself from losing control when she sees food.

She decides not to talk about eating or what others eat and not to be critical about the food. When you're at a party with people who focus on eating issues, it makes you feel anxious about your own eating. Part of the party plan is to be around people who are enjoying their food and the party, not people who are uptight about what they're eating.

Priorities form personal boundaries that protect by being a direct line to your intuition. An intuitive eater going to a party recognizes boundaries of her physical limits and the social stress, but still likes to have a good time. She handles this by acting dignified. This attitude puts people around her at ease.

When people are relaxed around you, they don't pressure you. The dignified way to control social stress is to maintain a cheerful, enthusiastic attitude that says, "I'm fine and having fun". This unconsciously let's others relax, which lets you relax and follow your plan. Ultimately you have fun at the party and importantly, you feel good about yourself the next day.

Counting calories is a personal priority that's no one's business but yours. If you join the spirit of the party without calling attention to the fact that not a bite of cake is passing your lips, no one will care.

People respond to attitude. President Ronald Regan was called the "teflon" president, possibly in part because he always projected a cheerful and enthusiastic attitude. Regan was also a great actor; sometimes we all have to put on a show.

Sometimes the only way to be dignified is to act dignified. If you aren't feeling dignified in your heart because the emotional baby wants to overeat, use the tool of tenacity to let your visual image and common sense weigh in. And then, something amazing happens: when you act dignified with the intention of respecting yourself, you become dignified! Trust your intuition and have fun.

Unless it is made clear in advance, a party is not a food orgy. 'Pigging out' is never really expected or respected. It signals misplaced emotional or social hunger.

Overeating:

- A person who quickly overeats may be afraid of missing something if he doesn't eat more. Perhaps this is the result of constant starvation. More likely it's an old self-defeating habit that has to be recognized, examined and discarded.

- A person may overeat at a party to avoid social interaction. It's impossible to carry on a conversation while you're stuffing your mouth with food. Some people use eating as a way to hide both socially and physically.

- A person may keep eating, going for seconds and thirds because he likes the attention of being fed. But this person obviously is not paying self-esteem or his body any attention. If so, he would recognize the beginnings of overeating indigestion. This sort of overeater's self-validation is dependent on the views of others. Eating to get attention is self-defeating. An attention-seeking eater is not respected by anyone and feels bad physically and emotionally after the party.

When practicing the attitude of dignity, you do not betray yourself with destructive behavior. To quit or give up is to betray yourself. To gorge means treating your body without respect, and that is self-betrayal. To starve yourself is equally a betrayal. There is no dignity in this behavior. There is only self-humiliation.

Dignity is not dependent on others. It doesn't matter what anyone thinks about your eating plan because no one is you. No one has your DNA, fingerprints, intuition or your life. When you feel dignified by your choices you feel complete.

Personal dignity is a powerful tool. Use it when eating alone or with others. Connecting with dignity brings the ability to cope better with storms and stress of life. It is dignified to reach out for others. It is dignified to ask for help. It is dignified to help yourself. It's about attitude.

"The only kind of dignity which is genuine is that which is not diminished by the indifference of others."[4] -- Dag Hammarskjold.

Dignity is held in place with tenacity. Intuitive eaters use the drive of tenacity to complete prudent choices with a positive, dignified attitude. Choosing to connect with your 6th sense embraces life from a place of dignity.

- Support comes from others in the form of admiration and respect. People will be attracted by your attitude. It will become easier to be in social environments without indulging in undignified eating.

- Dignity creates a gentle natural humility that's like charisma. Eating with dignity draws friends and family to join you.

- There is an inspirational and inclusive power in dignity that is easy to recognize. It feels good to be around dignified people. By showing this very personal level of self-respect, you inspire others to seek their own dignity.

- Dignity is a tool that helps you understand and honor who you are. You feel genuinely good about yourself when you understand how and what you need to eat to maintain your weight and quality of life.

Dignity is easy to recognize in others as an attitude of respect for their personal boundaries, a profound self-respect. Whether we like a person or not, whether we agree with a person or not, dignified behavior is always admired. Be that person. Be dignified.

Chapter 7: **Determination**

When confronted with eating challenges, determination kicks in to give insights that guide choices. For example, remember that oversized piece of birthday cake with the buttery icing on it and the jelly inside, or the second brownie, or bread and butter and potatoes? These sorts of challenges to self-control are easier to deal with when you use determination.

Before putting food in your mouth, determine:

- Is this going to give me energy?

- Is this going to make me feel good about myself?

- Is this smart to eat? Does it contain stuff my body won't respond to well?

- Is this what I want?

- Is this sabotage?

- Is this an emotional choice?

Choosing to eat food based on what you determine will protect you or give you pleasure, means you're in control of yourself. It's intuitive to love yourself and to fortify your life. Determination is the tool that affirms this.

Tap into the natural energy of determination and make a commitment to be intuitively satisfied with your eating choices.

"You've got to get up every morning with determination if you're going to go to bed with satisfaction."[1] George Lorimer

Determination is a power tool of intuitive eating that you can recognize as an energy or momentum. It's always present to use to help "power though" stressful eating situations. Acting with determination reinforces your commitment to listen to your gut instinct. The tool of determination is the right hand of your survival instinct.

We experience the energy and drive of determination physically, mentally and emotionally. When you're in sync with your best interests, determination is a force that will surround and protect you. For intuitive eaters, determination means not giving up! It's not an option.

If you're off-track, use the tool of determination along with honesty to practice a kind of 'tough love'. Use determination to examine your mental attitude and unmask dark places that are corruptions of your objective truth. Since what you think is based on what you remember, use determination to question yourself so you can stay clear about doing what's best. Using determination helps you separate your emotional need for attention from the physical need to eat. Intuitively recognizing your own self-deceptions sweeps them away.

Intuitive eating connects with gut determination. The intuitive eater sits down to eat and "sees" with his gut. He looks at food and uses the tough love of determination to see if it will enhance his health and his physique, or leave him feeling bloated and dissatisfied with himself. You know you're using determination when you feel the commitment to achieve your goal in every fiber of your being.

Chapter 8 : **Patience**

Patience is a stress buster. It's a tool of allowing and flexibility, and patience is a way of acknowledging effort. Our lives are busy. We're often on auto-drive, multi-tasking and under the gun. We're generally stressed, and so the idea of taking time to have patience may seem not relevant to your priorities. You may think, 'I don't have time to use this tool.' In fact nothing could be farther from the truth. Using patience when you eat is your intuitive key for reducing stress. Patience prevents abusive eating.

If you're not patient, you're abandoning yourself by ignoring your senses and dismissing your intuitive body connection. For example: daily stress triggers mindless eating. If you realize you're cramming food into your mouth before dinner, habit may be to punish yourself instead of recognizing a need to unwind. This attitude of impatience increases stress and leads to a cycle of destructive behavior. Patience is a stress buster because it gives you space to let go of useless and demanding habits.

"If you don't have time to do it right the first time,
when will you have time to do it over?"[1] John Wooden

A rigid habit of being hard on yourself creates resentment and is the opposite of having patience. Until you use the tool of patience, you may eat emotionally, miss a lot and generally sabotage yourself. Nobody can move forward to achieve their goals with resentment.

The process of patience begins with giving yourself credit for seeing what you're eating, tasting your food when you eat, listening to your body about its needs and responding to your body with respect.

Patience is the tool to count on to connect with your intuition, no matter how jammed, frustrated, exhausted or confused you are. It creates breathing space that gives perspective. As you learn to trust yourself around eating, you are able to relax and allow the natural process of trial and error to happen. You stay clear about eating priorities.

If you don't succeed at first, take a deep breath and try again; that's patience. Intuitive eating doesn't suddenly happen. It is a process of learning to connect with your senses and body, using your tools and trusting yourself.

Use patience to recognize:

- Your Body - including your five senses, is always communicating with you.

- Your Heart - beating to be heard and validated.

- Your Mind - holding your lessons learned.

- Spirit is experienced as passion, the joy of living, grief and wonder and is often referred to as the spark of life. Every person carries the spark of life. With patience, you can acknowledge and connect with it. The experience is glorious. Even when you ignore or deny it - it doesn't matter, because as long as you are alive, you have life.

Patience connects with your natural power of self-control. When you think of patience, remember to breathe. Breathing is a way of checking in with your body that balances body rhythms.

Patience is the cool tool because it connects with being relaxed and at peace with yourself. You digest food better and eat smarter when you're in harmony with yourself. As you fine tune input from the 5 senses, you recognize that you see, taste, hear and realize more and in this way patience becomes natural. Patience gives space to connect with your other tools.

To allow this important pause, you don't have to do anything extraordinary, just stay tuned to messages from your senses and observe yourself. Then, you can open your hand to let go of habits that are self-defeating.

- When a craving strikes, use patience to slowly deeply breathe in and out 3 times and count to 10 slowly. Then, step back from the moment to recognize what is driving you. Use prudence to decide options for dealing with an emotional issue in a way that makes you feel good about your choices.

Patience connects with and reinforces dignity. Without noticing, you are in control because you feel no stress. That's why patience is the cool tool.

When going out to eat, take time to really look with curiosity at the menu before ordering. Visualize and feed your perfect body. Be patient with your body and your desires. If having a hard time, use determination to focus and tenacity to reaffirm your choice to eat intuitively.

Let patience give you breathing space to open doors to your intuitive voice. Everything worth achieving takes patience including maintaining a healthy, energetic body. An important consistent difference between an intuitive eater and an emotional eater is: Intuitive eaters use the tool of patience every time they eat.

Patience is a form of empathy. Empathy is understanding and sharing feelings including your own. Notice when you're short with yourself around eating, such as when you're unforgiving over a food screw-up. There is often a surprising gap between what ought to have caused a screw up and what really did. Observe patiently and you'll recognize mental habits and your common sense. You'll know yourself better.

The next time a similar situation occurs, you can make a choice that feels good. Stuff happens. Patience gives you the fresh breath of another perspective.

Sometimes just one slight adjustment of furniture can change the way a room looks. This is the way patience works. Patience adjusts your perspective gently so you go from focusing with anxiety at mealtime to thinking about enjoying what you're eating.

Remember, we are people - not objects. Let the human connection of patience with yourself grow.

- Ultimately, patience is a form of compassion. Until you are compassionate with yourself, you cannot truly connect with your intuition.

- Being patient automatically makes you more comfortable in your own skin. The result is you are more alert and confident about making eating choices that achieve your goals.

- Patience relaxes your efforts with all of the intuitive tools to smooth the way. Use patience often to renew and refresh your intuitive connection.

Factoids:

- Bananas are the #1 fruit with the world's leading athletes. Bananas contain three natural sugars: sucrose, fructose and glucose combined with fiber. That's why bananas give instant sustained, substantial energy.

- Bananas also contain tryptophan which is a protein known to help us relax and feel happier, so slowly eat one for depression, SAD or to fight PMS.

- A banana is high in iron which can help prevent some cases of anemia. It is extremely high in potassium but low in salt, so the US Food and Drug Administration promotes eating bananas to reduce the risk of high blood pressure. According to the New England Journal of Medicine, bananas can reduce the risk of death by strokes by as much as 40%.[7]

- Eat a banana when stressed because potassium helps to normalize your heartbeat, regulate water balance and control blood sugar levels. Bananas help regain balance and that feeling of control.

- This same potassium gives brainpower by sending oxygen to your brain, making you more alert, according to research done with students. Keep a stash of bananas to keep yourself mentally fresher.

- It's said the high fiber in bananas helps maintain normal bowel movements.

- Try curing a hangover with a banana milkshake, adding a teaspoon of honey. The milk soothes and re-hydrates, the banana will help calm the stomach, while the honey replaces depleted blood sugar levels.

- Bananas can have a natural anti-acid effect, reducing irritation by coating the lining of the stomach and relieving heartburn. Because of their soft texture and smoothness, people with ulcers can eat bananas.[2]

- Bananas are easily available, give energy, are good for health and can help overcome eating challenges. Bananas are an amazing food!

Am I Really Hungry?

Chapter 9 : Foresight

Foresight keeps you clear about the present, which helps you stay emotionally grounded around eating. Foresight is looking ahead at the consequences of what you're about to do. For example, foresight is looking both ways before you cross the street.

Using foresight at mealtime:

- Prepares you for the unexpected.

- Connects with a sense of purpose when you eat, which is to get energy through nourishment and feel good while you enjoy your meal.

- Enables balance in action and goals by keeping you in touch with the present.

- Creates clarity of choices by combining the perspective of dignity with the reality of your moment.

- Is the tool of intuitive self-defense that you can always tap into using the tool of patience.

"May you have the hindsight to know where you've been, the foresight to know where you are going, and the insight to know when you have gone too far." Irish Saying

This quote is saying:

- Hindsight is prudence.

- Foresight is staying connected to the moment.

- And Insight is the result of experience.

Foresight connects with what you sense, feel and think. It is the 360-degree "now". Observe and nourish yourself with foresight. This is a great habit. As you fine-tune with foresight, cravings will change.

Typically we think of foresight as planning ahead. Planning ahead makes life easier when based on intuitive needs. Shopping with foresight brings healthy, nourishing meaningful food into your home.

When grocery shopping with foresight:

- Listen to your body to connect with your needs.

- Keep a running list of what you need. Read it before shopping and know the quality of what you buy using common sense and experience.

- Only buy what's on your list.

- Use your senses before you put anything in the basket.

  - Eyes see what's quality and what will defeat your goals.

  - Ears hear about what's fresh, what's a bargain, or misleading.

  - Touch and smell recognize if something is old or fresh.

When going out to dinner, have something healthy earlier to take the edge off. Eat an apple or have a small bowl of oatmeal. This way you won't be so hungry that you order more than your body really need.

By eating a snack in advance, you'll be more physically relaxed and more social. I always do this. It takes the urgency off of my hunger so I order prudently and enjoy the social experience of going out more.

> *"There are three constants in life… change, choice, and principles."*[1] *Stephen R. Covey*

Use curiosity along with foresight to break out of rigid eating patterns formed since you were born. Today is the beginning of the rest of your life. Use patience to be flexible and prudent. When you listen to your body about what you want to eat, it can be quite surprising. Surprise yourself.

Every day is an opportunity to get in touch with your unique body rhythms. Each organ must be nourished to thrive. Every seven years each cell in your body is entirely new. Although you seem to be the same old self, you're feeding a much younger body.

When you eat at home, practice flexibility by allowing yourself to eat anything you want that's nourishing, even if it's steak for breakfast and scrambled eggs at night. Let foresight connect you with what makes sense for your body.

Use curiosity to experiment and tenacity to stay committed to eating goals. Try having peanut butter on a bagel for breakfast. Put just one tablespoon on each half. You will discover that you won't be hungry for hours because peanut butter takes longer to digest than butter or cheese.

Foresight keeps you clear about the present. Being clear about needs and desires in the present means you can respond to your best advantage and plan wisely for the future. Use foresight to protect yourself from impulses and circumstances that are self-destructive.

When you eat, you are doing much more than getting energy for the next day. You are laying the foundation for your future. Foresight pays off when you least expect it!

Factoids:

Don't stock up with cookies, candy or chips in your home. Make it inconvenient to have these mindless nibbles.

- Instead, keep unsweetened frozen blueberries, strawberries, blackberries or raspberries in the freezer for sweet noshing. Berries taste good, are easy to handle and have antioxidants and fiber. You can buy unsweetened frozen cantaloupes or mangos to have on hand, too. I also like to freeze seedless grapes and then enjoy them as a cool snack.

- Mix any frozen fruit with your favorite yogurt for a fruit smoothie. If your yogurt is flavored, it already has a sweetener in it. Think about your choices with the tool of prudence and stay connected to your dignity when you snack.

- If you want to eat fruit plain, try to develop a taste for the natural flavor. If you find it bitter, add a scant teaspoon of honey or other sweetener. Taste preferences are something we learn. Tune into what your body really wants instead of what you "think" you like. Use the tool of curiosity to experiment and get to know yourself better.

Am I Really Hungry?

Chapter 10 : **Self-Discipline**

Intuitive eaters use self-discipline as a tool to overcome disappointment. It is an intuitive way of giving yourself support and guidance. This guidance provides the stability we all need to cope with the zig-zag path of life.

Self-discipline is a kind of self-respect. It is not a way of criticizing. Self-discipline is a tool you can count on to guide you forward with body and life goals.

Think of self-discipline like a railing along a steep flight of stairs. You hold onto the railing to keep balanced as you navigate the way. Use this tool to stay on your eating path. Rather than listen to a chorus of peer pressure or the emotional lure of your thoughts or inner dialogue when you sit down to eat, self-discipline is the power tool intuitive eaters use to follow what feels right. This is being self-reliant.

"Nothing can bring you peace but yourself.
Nothing can bring you peace but the triumph of principles."[1]
Ralph Waldo Emerson

Self-discipline is the opposite of passing judgment about yourself. Non-judgmental means trusting your intuitive voice and responding to your whole self with dignity.

When you eat with self-discipline you experience:

- Less stress: because self-discipline is a form of intuitive confidence that feels like self-reliance. As you use the tools, you are confident in your choices, and therefore, feel in harmony with your body. The result is you relax when eating which means you eat slower, enjoy food more and digest it better. It also means you are less likely to overeat.

- Personal comfort: because self-discipline is a way of protecting yourself. Eating with the tools of prudence, patience and dignity is like having a safety net guiding you. You feel taken care of.

- Ease about your body: because you know you are a work in progress. Patience tells you this. See your perfect body in your mind and let intuition guide you to nurture it. Instead of being in a power struggle with your body, trust foresight to bring your physicality in sync with your mental image.

Because life is constantly changing, intuitive self-discipline is constantly responding and developing. Curiosity and dignity help you maintain a flexible attitude with yourself. Use intuitive tools to lean on and connect with self-discipline. When you have perspective, it becomes obvious that self-discipline puts a personal stamp on everything you do.

"Every job is a self-portrait of the person who did it.
Autograph your work with excellence." anon

As you use self-discipline, you will meet the part of yourself that brings rewarding surprise, pleasure and a sense of accomplishment. Try it.

Chapter 11 : **Courage**

Courage propels you through obstacles strewn along your path. It's a kind of intuitive glue that holds you together when times get rough.

- Every change you make is an act of courage. This includes changing your approach to eating, changing your ideas or changing your habits.

- It takes courage to believe in yourself and not cave to peer pressure to eat or do or be who you are not.

- It takes courage to resist temptation created by old emotional habits and to stand strong for your choices. Ah yes, here again is that incredibly delectable piece of birthday cake and this time it's sitting with a bowl of butter pecan ice cream. It takes courage, determination and prudence to honor yourself. It's courage that helps you stick to your resolve.

Courage is incomparable energy you're born with. It's the intuitive lifeline you can always opt for. The energy of courage is a boldness that feels like enthusiasm with backbone. It is the diamond point of the arrow of your intuition. Courage is an intimate part of your inner strength, fortified by clarity of what is right. For this reason, courage is the ultimate enhancer of all your intuitive tools.

"Courage is not simply one of the virtues,
but the form of every virtue at the testing point."[1] C.S. Lewis

Feelings of courage come naturally to us as young children and then are dampened by rebuffs, put downs or other unpleasant real experiences. As you learn to be subservient to peer pressure, to rules that may not make sense, to traditions that are so old no one remembers how they started, and as you learn to ignore your intuitive voice, you learn to put a lid on your innate courage and give power to fear.

While the experience of fear is real, courage balanced with prudence is your intuitive realization that there are other things more important in your life than fear. Fine-tuning your senses and intuitive tools reconnects you with your natural lifeline of personal courage.

Courage helps you stick to your resolve:

- It keeps you determined.

- It gives you patience.

- It is always available.

You have access to the tool of courage 24/7 - wear it.

".. screw your courage to the sticking-place. And we'll not fail."[2]
Lady Macbeth, Shakespeare

Using the tools of courage and dignity to do the right thing when you're all alone with a quart of ice cream is intuitive eating. It takes courage to make the right choice at a party when you are surrounded by well-meaning friends and it always takes courage to laugh when you're discouraged or afraid. When you tap into your courage, nutritional choices get easier.

Media shows courageous acts that are super-hero brazen but in fact, courage is ultimately a very private choice you make alone. Making difficult or unpleasant choices because you feel they are right is very courageous. Every day you make choices that are courageous.

Courage is as natural as breathing. You began life with courage mainlining your natural enthusiasm and that is how you are meant to live. As you learn to protect yourself by respecting yourself and reconnecting with your inborn courage, it's exciting.

"Courage is what it takes to stand up and speak;

courage is also what it takes to sit down and listen."[3]
Winston Churchill

Chapter 12 : **The 10th Tool**

This 10th tool is revealed in Chapter 18. The first 9 must be chewed, swallowed and digested first. Nutritionists say that until you process food by digesting it, your body cannot absorb benefit from eating. It's time to learn to enjoy and master the art of eating. Then you will be ready to digest the mystery tool.

The 10th tool is a tape that holds together your intuitive perspective so that it shines through all life's challenges. This tool works like a beam of light. You will recognize it instantly. Curiosity about this is healthy. In the silent process of "curious thinking," your senses connect with your mind. In fact, we do a lot of "curious thinking" without realizing it. This is good because there are a lot of real things to think about.

Your chest of intuitive tools is a protective arsenal that filters confusion about eating to give the insight of clarity. Use the tools to maintain and sustain your ideal weight. They are light to carry and natural to use. The tools work together, effectively guiding you toward a renewed level of connection with your 6th sense. The result is satisfaction with your body and with yourself.

Quick Tool Summary:

- Foresight / self-defense
- Patience / breathing room
- Curiosity / my 5 senses and my mind
- Prudence / my options
- Tenacity / commitment to myself
- Dignity / self-respect
- Determination / follow through
- Self-discipline / my intuition
- Courage / my lifeline
- ????? / personal forgiveness

Am I Really Hungry?

Chapter 13 : **Transformational Eating / The Shift**

"It takes a lot of courage to release the familiar and seemingly secure, to embrace the new. But there is no real security in what is no longer meaningful. There is more security in the adventurous and exciting, for in movement there is life, and in change there is power."[1] Alan Cohen

Transformation means a thorough or dramatic change. It's radical to stop thinking of yourself as a 'dieter'. This transformation is you de-programming and re-routing your thinking. With practice, you go from feeling restrained by diet plans and calorie requirements to trusting your own judgment.

Transforming from a dieter into an intuitive eater is big. It's like being a caterpillar and becoming a butterfly. The caterpillar eats and weaves her cocoon of change instinctively. There is no inner dialogue challenging, so she eats for energy and life. Because dieters are accustomed to letting inner dialogue challenge and dictate what to do with their bodies, this transformation takes more effort.

Eating focused on a strict system or pattern is an intuitive disconnect because it ignores messages from your body. Begin your transformation by connecting with your 5 senses to notice your body. Really look at food when you think about eating it. Notice if it has an aroma. If you had it before, remember what it tastes like. *Don't think - Remember with your senses.*

When you eat, physically and emotionally you need food for energy and strength. Intuition coordinates hunger urges so that what you want is what you need. Depend on the tools for balanced choices. You will know you are using all 6 senses when you feel in sync with yourself.

When all 6 senses are clearly in the present, you have a new awareness. Courage feels like backbone and foresight protects you. Patience opens up the eating experience and dignity gives self-control that leads to wise choices.

Intuition is your inner 'GPS' navigating the best way to get where you want to go. Use it to reshape your body and revolutionize your eating perspective. Ultimately the path of opportunity, the sum of your potential, is always available. That's what this transformation is about.

Transforming includes learning to focus on one meal at a time. Planning dinner while eating lunch means before one meal is digested, you are mentally eating again! This is not intuitive. No other living creature does it. Instinct is to eat just enough and trust hunger will return and another meal will be found. It's intuitive to focus on and appreciate what you eat while you're eating it.

Using curiosity, invisible habits that don't serve you become obvious. You can ride out invisible habits and forget them. Curiosity guides you to notice what you eat while patience, determination and tenacity wear away habits and dignity maintains your priorities.

Invisible self-defeating eating habits that are not intuitive include:

- focusing on food days in advance of eating
- thinking about calories instead of quality or need
- labeling everything to do with eating as 'good' or 'bad'

According to Jay Dixit (Sr. Editor, Psychology Today, when changing eating habits, *"The hardest part is the first 72 hours when eating right is an act of will. After two or three weeks of sticking to it, your hunger and cravings subside, and control over eating choices becomes automatic. ... Breaking out of your routine may make you more aware of your choices in general and less likely to engage in mindless eating."*[2]

Honesty

The top requirement for eating intuitively is honesty with yourself around food and eating. Honesty means no rationalizing or justifying. It includes keeping an open mind, and being tenacious about using the tools. Because honesty is the compass in your intuitive tool chest, it always points to the right choice, which is your intuitive truth.

When you are unsure about an eating choice, use uncompromising, pitiless honesty. This keeps you clear about truth and that is the power base of your self-control.

Being an intuitive eater will not become routine because every time you eat is a new perspective. Each meal is the opportunity for you to make fresh eating choices.

What to do:

- Slow down and smell the coffee. Remember to be honest and respect yourself.

- Recognize what you see, hear, taste, smell and touch.

- Notice what's on your plate.

- Intuitive tools will override counter-intuitive input from your mind or emotions.

For example:

You're served a large plate overflowing with delicious food. Your mind says, it's so good, why not eat it all? Emotionally you want to fill up on something good. But your senses - which protect your body - see, smell, taste and feel gluttony with its side effects of sluggishness, intestinal problems and personal disappointment. Use patience to connect with your body and take a deep breath in and out.

Intuition might gently suggest you ask for a smaller plate and then serve yourself from the initial plate and have the remainder either packed for take-out or returned to the kitchen.

As you transform to eating intuitively, remember the senses are passive and can easily be ignored. If you don't pay attention you can easily close your eyes, block out the sound of someone's voice, hold your nose, get past your gag reflex, ignore getting burned by the sun or put that little voice on hold.

The result of ignoring your 6 senses is a disconnect from yourself, which means making wrong connections and wrong decisions. Things just don't feel right. That feeling is intuition telling you, you're off-track.

Intuitive eating looks at the big picture at mealtime. It balances what you sense physically with messages from your mind and emotions. All of these are equally important parts of who you are and keep you tuned-in to eating exactly what your body needs.

Eating Journal

Download a FREE *Am I Really Hungry?* journal page from IntuEating.com and see an example at the back of this book.

A food journal is helpful in transforming because it's a way of connecting with being truthful with yourself. Keeping a journal for four weeks identifies invisible eating habits. If you decide to download the journal, then I suggest instead of listing what you eat at each meal, take a photo with your phone and download it to your journal page. Seeing it is powerful.

When Journaling:

- Write down your eating goals. Remember you're now in transition from a dieter to an intuitive eater. Your goals are related to quality of life and feeling in sync with your body instead of your weight.

- Stay connected with intuitive tools as you make eating choices.

- Start with this one goal: Promise yourself to use curiosity to learn about what you eat before taking a bite, by paying attention with your senses, including common sense.

After you eat or snack, write it in the journal with details:

- My Food Choices: be detailed, be honest or take a photo for your records

- Location: learn if you eat at your desk, in the car or at the table

- My Hunger: connect with your body to see if you eat because of stress or habit or wait until you are ravenous to recognize signals from your body

- My Feelings: connect with your whole self; are you stressed or distracted while eating? Do you enjoy meals?

- Self-Control: notice what you notice; when using your intuition self-control feels natural. Are you struggling with your choices, slipping, falling off the wagon? Observing yourself changes the way you do things.

- What intuitive tools am I using? Rely on the tools and your senses.

- Notes/Thoughts- write whatever comes to mind

After two weeks, review your journal to notice habits you want to lose like waiting to feel ravenous before feeding yourself, or eating mindlessly while watching TV or you may notice you eat more when you eat out. Some people discover they skip meals only to, unfortunately, splurge later.

Use curiosity to connect with your senses and messages from your body. Be a detective: Identify foods that make you feel sluggish or those that don't feel good an hour later, foods that fill you up for a while and those that keep you fueled, so that you can choose wisely.

Learn from reading your journal about habits you want to acquire, like using foresight before ordering to connect with prudence when deciding eating choices, and connecting with tenacity before beginning to eat. This is you intuitively pulling it all together to make the most of your life. All of us work through problems we are unaware of. Be kind to yourself.

Finally, notice tools you use most. Courage, tenacity, dignity and patience are the top four mentioned by dieters as helpful for keeping perspective and making the transformation.

Transformational eating is going from a place of non-productive habits to a stream of synchronicity. When you're clear about intuitive tools, it is natural to let them work for you. This is a gentle process that evolves with patience and persistence. Ultimately you transform your attitude, levels of enjoyment and physical appearance.

Your body is designed to maximize the amount of energy you get from foods which means intuitively, you are very good at selecting food that is good for you. Becoming an intuitive eater happens gradually. Being in sync with yourself feels like being in the flow, being in rhythm with your world and yourself. It is the power of self-control over what you do with your body, yourself and your life.

Factoids:

- Intuitive eating shifts weight management from a challenge to a natural lifestyle.

- Focusing on enjoying food as a way of nourishing your body and getting the most out of life, rewires thinking so your brain connects self-respect, courage, prudence and tenacity with your body. It's part of the transformation.

- Look at your meal and think, 'I'm going to feel great after I eat this.'

Chapter 14: Hunger- **What is it? How can I recognize it? What does it mean?**

"Before you take another step, step back into yourself.
If you can govern yourself and be your own master, yours is the
whole wide world and everything within it."[1] Paul Fleming

Intuition connects your whole being: body, mind, and heart. A fancy word for this way of looking at the whole picture of who you are is "holistic". The word: *holistic* sounds like the word: *whole.* Intuition is the natural holistic intrapersonal link that connects your mental, emotional and physical needs so that you can know what you're hungry for.

There are 4 kinds of hunger. All are easily confused with physical hunger. Knowing why you feel hungry and what you are hungry for is as important as realizing when you are hungry.

4 Types of Hunger:

Physical hunger: is your genuine bodily need. It is satisfied by eating nourishing food, not by junk food or the 'wrong' food. Although foods with no nutritional value may have bulk, they do not satisfy physical hunger. Your body wants and needs more.

- **Physical signs of bodily hunger include:**

    growls

    pangs

    hollow feelings in your stomach

    n.b. Nat'l
    cf. Hygiene

- **Mental signs of bodily hunger include:**

    fogginess

    lack of concentration

    headache

    short temper

    fatigue

Emotional hunger: Emotions often trigger abusive eating. Emotional eating can be a response, a defense or even habit, with no connection to your nutritional needs. It's often a reaction to loneliness, anger, emptiness, happiness, guilt, fear or stress. Emotional hunger can be satisfied by play, touch, nature, romance, music, art, love and excitement. When satisfied emotionally, people often forget about food and are instead 'high on life'.

Mental hunger: includes psychological, intellectual, social or habitual hunger. It is satisfied by conversation, hobbies, entertainment, reading, playing games for fun. Sharing the passion of play can consume your attention to the point of forgetting to eat. Even casual encounters have an impact on satisfying this appetite. When not satisfied, mental hunger can trigger emotional eating.

Intuitive hunger: is the desire for clarity, balance and protection because these are the source of success, excitement, comfort and inner peace.

To satisfy this:

- Be honest with yourself, use patience and respond to what you sense.

- Listen to that little voice when you 'feel' like overindulging.

- Let yourself feel determination and connect with prudence.

"Just as food is needed for the body, love is needed for the soul."[2]
Osho

It's natural to enjoy food. What makes food enjoyable besides taste, is understanding what it does for your life. The food you eat is an investment in your future. Sometimes eating is like taking medicine because your body needs a nutriment to be healthy. Sometimes a food will give your skin a glow or give you a night sleep. Using curiosity keeps you aware of food that feels good and food that doesn't.

"Let food be thy medicine, and medicine be thy food." Hippocrates

Intuitive tools, working with the 5 senses, keep clear where hunger is coming from. You can recognize if hunger is caused by stress, frustration or physical need. When you know why you're hungry, you know what to eat to feel satisfied.

Without intuitive connections to understand the source of hunger, internal traffic jams that feel like confusion occur. Confusion leads to unhealthy habits.

Self-destructive habits:

- Obsessing about food makes you think you're physically hungry when you're not. Obsessing is often a reaction to emotional stress. As a result, you may feed loneliness or stress with cookies.

- Eating pre-planned meals can feel restrictive and doesn't relate to actual physical hunger at mealtime, which creates confusion. If you like to pre-plan because it's comforting, please allow yourself the tool of curiosity and be flexible. If the planned food doesn't excite your senses, then make another prudent choice that clearly feels right.

"If you don't know when you're hungry, you don't know when you're full, so you won't know when to stop eating."[10] Elisabetta Politi, RD, Duke University Diet &Fitness Center

Discover yourself. It's common to underestimate amount when eating is reactive or a habit. Use curiosity and be honest with yourself.

- If you have trouble being clear about what you're eating, keep a food journal to help break a cycle of food denial.

- If you believe you're overeating, instead of having dessert, at the end of the meal, take that time to write down what you just ate. Then, get curious about how you feel, and think about how you chose what you ate. You might be surprised.

"Eat breakfast like a king, lunch like a prince and dinner like a pauper."[4] Adelle Davis

Hunger is personal. Experiment to see what satisfies you. Everyone has unique hunger cycles and body rhythms. Some people are hungriest in the morning. Some learn that a big midday meal is the most satisfying time to eat and some prefer to eat their largest meal at night. Others eat a bunch of small-snack sized meals throughout the day. Eating is a personal choice and private need.

Social pressure can place us in eating environments when we are not physically hungry. Self-discipline and dignity help when physical need runs contrary to social pressures.

In an awkward social situation where you're not hungry:

- Be gracious and respectful of others.
- Don't talk about eating or food because this may make you and others uncomfortable.
- Commit to your choice and trust that you'll eat when you need to. Be dignified.
- Enjoy the company and enjoy what you eat.
- Be flexible.
- Order a small salad and eat very slowly.
- Don't feel obligated to finish by cleaning your plate.
- Enjoy the social experience of sharing a meal. Use courage.
- Use foresight to modify eating during the day so you can enjoy a dinner party.
- Eat small but nutritionally satisfying portions. As long as you're comfortable with yourself, everyone else will be too.
- If someone makes a negative comment about your diet, smile and say you are following your intuition. No one can argue with that.

State of Mind

You can recognize hunger through your state of mind. Our state of mind reflects pressures and realities. You may be preoccupied, happy, sad, bored, excited, worried, etc. Since a state of mind is always in flux, keeping your senses finely tuned when you think you're hungry keeps you in the present so that non-related issues are kept at bay. Use intuitive tools to cut through mental distractions and recognize the source of hunger.

Although intuitive eaters say they do not "diet", they 'watch' everything they eat. Before eating, they observe themselves, how their body feels and what's on the table. By using tools first, good choices kick in 'automatically'. An open, flexible state of mind determines food choices.

Using foresight for self-defense identifies emotional distractions that feel like hunger. There is an expression: 'To be forewarned is to be forearmed.' This means using foresight can control the impact of stress on your eating. Foresight gives you the advantage of perspective.

Emotional hot buttons are often reactions to mental distractions. Mental distractions are thoughts mostly coming from inner dialogue. These are usually harsh personal criticisms based on insecurity and create irrational self-judgment.

To deal with mind distractions and triumph over inner dialogue:

- Notice what 's creating the inner dialogue.

- Use tenacity along with common sense to stay clear about eating for energy and health. Focusing on physical reality gives less significance to emotional stuff or mental distractions.

- Use prudence to consider eating options.

- Use patience to sabotage stress and create a comfort zone that feels like self control.

- This brings courage and clarity to your mental state. You feel a light sense of relief as you reconnect with yourself.

- Self-respect recognizes the difference between inner voice and inner dialogue.

- Tenacity along with determination guides choices for intuitive eating. You feel good. Goodbye inner dialogue.

When you feel hungry, use curiosity.

- What is my state of mind?

- Why do I feel hungry?

- Is it a response to my body or my emotions?

- Is it a response to stress?

- What am I really hungry for?

- How will my body feel if I eat now?

Recognizing physical symptoms of hunger takes effort until it becomes automatic. You may realize that you aren't hungry, or you'll realize a meal you're considering will feel bad an hour later, or you might decide the perfect meal is on your plate. Notice what you notice. Depend on your senses to tune into your body. Really see what you're eating and make an effort to be aware of how you feel. Learn about yourself.

Use tenacity. Since the stomach is directly connected with the mind and emotions, tenacity can determine: "Am I hungry or do I just think it's time to eat?" or "Does my body want that wonderful double chocolate brownie or that second cheeseburger, or am I feeding an emotional need?"

Think out of the box when eating doesn't satisfy physical hunger. Intuitive tools, especially prudence and dignity, help. The tools help you recognize what's pushing you to eat because they tune you into yourself. Observing hunger with the tools of patience, determination and self-respect creates the courage to make prudent eating choices and feel confident physically and emotionally.

"Whether you think you can or whether you think you can't, you're right."[5] *Henry Ford*

We eat to replace energy. Burning calories is using energy. Everything you do burns calories - even eating or reading this book. Every effort you put into discovering your habits and connecting with your senses and using your intuitive tools, burns calories.

Use courage and be bold. Take control of food choices by trying new foods. Two things can happen that might surprise you. You might enjoy the new food and you might feel your hunger satisfied. Learning about yourself is intuitive. It is part of the process of patience. Patience allows trial and error. The result is satisfaction.

Two Kinds of Cravings:

- Unhealthy craving: can mean junk food or be mistaken as comfort food. The hunger is not physical so there is little or no nutritional benefit. An effective method for killing this sort of craving is the quote below. If you do this the next time you're craving a quart of ice cream, it will probably stop before you swallow:

"..imagine yourself eating something you would like to stop eating, and then imagine something repulsive (like maggots wiggling around in it) happening while you're eating the food"[6] Jon Gabriel

- Intuitive craving: occurs when you are really in tune with yourself physically, mentally and emotionally. The hint that it's intuitive is that this type of craving is never destructive or self-abusive in any way. When you eat what you intuitively crave, you feel good about it an hour later.

Hunger and Sleep:

Have you ever been unable to sleep because your stomach was keeping you awake? It's really uncomfortable isn't it? By connecting with your body when you eat, you will sleep better.

Using the senses includes using common sense. Common sense is intuition that clearly serves your best interest. If your body regularly wakes up in the middle of the night because you're hungry, it's time to step out of the box of sleep-assisting drugs and pay attention to messages you're getting in the middle of the night. Foresight, tenacity and self-discipline can help you rest.

It's easy to confuse hunger with stress. Stress triggers the hunger hormone, ghrelin. This was discovered by research done on why people who are stressed or depressed tend to overeat.

Ghrelin is related to our survival instinct and acts like intuition because it doesn't just relate to the stomach but in fact, is a hormone that reflects the mind, senses and mood. When Dr. Lutter says in the quote below this hormone coordinates an entire behavioral response, he is saying it affects us holistically.

Dr. Michael Lutter, instructor of psychiatry at UT Southwestern and lead author of the study (on ghrelin), said,

"Our findings support the idea that these hunger hormones don't do just one thing; rather, they coordinate an entire behavioral response to stress and probably affect mood, stress and energy levels."

"However, this new research suggests that if you block ghrelin signaling, you might actually increase anxiety and depression, which would be bad," Dr. Zigman said.

Until modern times, the one common human experience was securing enough food to prevent starvation. Our hunter-gatherer ancestors needed to be as calm and collected as possible when it was time to venture out in search of food, or risk becoming dinner themselves, Dr. Zigman said, adding that the anti-anxiety effects of hunger-induced ghrelin may have provided a survival advantage."[7]

Since this feeling of hunger doesn't relate to a nutritional need, it's natural that experiencing it causes confusion. The point is that while ghrelin may trigger a feeling of hunger, it doesn't mean you need to eat. Instead, hunger caused by stress means you need to get to the root of your stress and feed it with realistic physical, emotional or mental nourishment. You can do this. Trust your senses and trust yourself.

Stress and Sleep:

Whatever is keeping you up at night will still be on your mind when you wake up in the morning. Our brain works even when we're asleep. Knowing this gives "permission" to let go of stress at night because you need to sleep and can trust your brain will wake up with something. Connect with intuition using tenacity, determination and patience to relax. When stress is keeping you up, say to yourself: "I am letting go of my stress now so that I can sleep. When I wake up, I will feel refreshed and strong to deal with my day." Keep repeating it and close your eyes.

If you wake up at night feeling that eating solution to help you sleep, think again. Clearly you will not starve to death overnight. Imagine letting go of the feeling. Visualize your limbs sinking into the bed, and imagine a place where you are at utter peace. Close your eyes and see it. Repeat, "I am letting go of my stress now so that I can sleep. When I wake up, I will feel refreshed and strong to deal with my day." Breathe deeply for several minutes; the feeling of hunger will pass and sleep will come.

It is common to confuse hunger with thirst. Sometimes thirst wakes me up with a weird taste in my mouth. For this reason, I keep a glass of water by my bed. Before I go to sleep, I put 1/2 teaspoon of apple cider vinegar in the glass of water. This gives it a kind of gentle cleansing taste - not as acidic as lemon. If I wake up craving something in my stomach, I drink a few swallows of water and then lay back down. The cider water cleans the taste in my mouth, satisfies my urge and I fall back to sleep.

According to the Harvard Health Letter, restless nights are often the result of indigestion or constipation that we are unaware of. Gas discomfort caused by incomplete digestion or swallowing air can cause restless sleep. Curiosity, the tool of observation, clues you into what may cause gas or incomplete digestion.

- Do I chew before swallowing?

- Do I talk while I'm eating?

- Do I gulp down my food?

Popular tips to avoid gas:

- Avoid carbonated drinks.

- Limit sugar and alcohol.

- Limit gas producing foods such as cauliflower, brussel sprouts, peas, beans, lentils and cabbage.

- Consuming excess fiber can create the feeling we call bloat.

Chew slowly, talk less, chew more. Taste your food. Eat slowly so that the natural process of digestion can occur. The body is efficient but not robotic. Digestion begins with chewing. Not only is food broken down so that its nutritional content is more available, but there are natural enzymes in saliva which prepare food for your stomach. Digestion is not instant. Learn about your body.

I have learned that alcohol keeps me awake. Sometimes I forget about this when I'm out enjoying a drink, and I pay later. Some people find dairy products hard to digest and will keep away from them in the evening. Digestion is personal, so we each need to connect with curiosity and use tenacity to recognize what works for our body.

"Pay attention to your body. The point is that every body is different. You have to figure out what works for you."[8]
Andrew Weil, MD

As you recognize patterns, you can change them. You can tune into hunger with mind, heart and body to see where it comes from and intuitively recognize habits that don't maintain your healthy weight.

Nutrition:

A natural result of a well-nourished body is a good night's sleep. Nourishment does not always mean food. You are nourished by conversation, music, laughter, kindness, success, friendship plus many other ways that naturally occur. All have a profound impact on comfort with yourself, which means all of types of nourishment have an impact upon perceived hunger. Because nourishment is the source of a healthy body, mind and spirit, intuitive eaters seek it.

Eating Habits:

The word habit immediately conjures up mindless eating. Eating habits can cause weight gain. A habit is something you do without thinking about it. This is not healthy eating. Eating habits are a modern dilemma.

In the "old days" people were forced to eat a variety of foods based on what was seasonally available. This was better for nourishing the body because variety means feeding your body different vitamins, enzymes, and minerals throughout the year. Variety makes sure that different organs get what they need to regenerate cells. Cravings, as we know them, didn't exist. Eating habits are not naturally good for you.

Comfort Foods:

Associated with nostalgia, comfort foods are a personal choice. It's not the food, it's the quantity consumed and the timing around eating that impacts sleeping or weight gain. If your favorite comfort food is grandma's chicken soup and you have this for dinner, then it's nourishing and comforting. If you have a bowl of chicken soup at 3am, it may keep you awake. If comfort food is a sweet like ice cream, then moderation makes sense. Also, eating a bowl of ice cream at night will keep many people up because it can create gas and bloating.

No matter how old you are, every day you are feeding a hungry new body. The only reason why we behave our birth age is because special cells in the brain endure from birth to death. Every other cell in our body lives a unique life cycle.

Every 5 days the lining of the stomach is new, and skin is recycled every 2 weeks. The liver, which is the filter system of poisons that pass our lips, has a turnover time of about once a year and even bones endure non-stop makeover. In adults, the entire skeleton is new every 10 years. Wow!

Imagine your body is new and see your ideal healthy body. This is your goal. This is the body you maintain. When you feed a body you love and see as ideal, you relate to hunger and yourself differently. It's liberating.

"Whatever your age, your body is many years younger. In fact, even if you're middle aged, most of you may be just 10 years old or less."[9] Dr. Jonas Frisen

Factoids:

- The body is always replacing cells, which means internal nourishment needs constantly vary. Physical hunger will nudge relentlessly when your body needs any element of nutrition. It could be as obvious as protein or as obscure as a trace mineral deficiency.

- If you're still hungry after a meal, it may be that the meal didn't satisfy you physically. It doesn't mean you need to eat more of the same food. For example, you eat a hamburger and fries for dinner and are still hungry. Having another hamburger, even without the bun, is not the answer. It may be something as simple as eating a pickle or you may be thirsty. Consider your options.

- When physically hungry, the feeling doesn't go away if you wait it out. If emotionally hungry, often doing something besides eating satisfies your real need and the craving disappears.

- The Cornell University Food and Brand Lab has a great website. It includes a helpful "Tip Sheet" that talks about everything from comfort food habits, to buying in bulk, to relationships between taking certain pills and eating, to changing your family's eating habits. Knowing these things helps you keep eating priorities straight. Check it out: http://foodpsychology.cornell.edu/tipsheet.htm

- It's best not to eat any food closer than 2 hours before you go to sleep. The stomach needs time to digest food. Digesting food burns energy. Since many foods such as bread, meat and vegetables are not in the form where our body can get nourishment from them as soon as you eat them, hormones and enzymes in your body break down (digest) your food so that you can receive nourishment. This is an active process.

- Sometimes after a large meal you may feel a desire to rest, but this doesn't signal sleep. Digestion and sleep are not designed to occur at the same time in your body. A good night's sleep occurs after the work of digestion is complete.

- The body digests food and turns it into energy. If you are sleep deprived, your digestion process may be out of whack. Sleeping is when our body most efficiently restores energy.

- Food is fuel and sleep is the battery that recharges your body so you can use it. You can have a full tank but feel tired if you need to recharge. Instead of overeating, try a power nap for 10 to 30 minutes for the boost that sparks.

- I like pickles and was able to look up the nutrition facts for eating one pickle on: **http://www.nutritiondata.com/** This useful website for practicing the tool of curiosity states that one pickle spear is a good source of vitamin A, potassium, manganese, dietary fiber, vitamin K and calcium. I discovered pickles are anti-inflammatory. At the same time, I learned they can be high in sodium. Besides nutritional information, this site provides easy to use tools for comparing nutritional content of foods.

Am I Really Hungry?

Chapter 15 : **Frustration**

Frustration is an intuitive message. The purpose is to create action. Just like you see without looking and hear without listening, you experience frustration automatically. This confused, unpleasant feeling signals a need for change. Sometimes it's a gentle persistent tap on the shoulder and sometimes it's a slap across the face.

Feeling frustrated around eating is a signal to use your senses and intuitive tools to reconnect with your whole self. Doing this resets priorities and begins momentum to overcome what is causing the frustration.

Often, eating and weight management frustration signals fear you may be unable to control your eating. Deep down the fear is that you cannot trust yourself. This is a dark feeling and it stings. Fortunately, intuitive tools give a lifeline and direction to lean into and depend on when you're frustrated.

When my cousin Linda, a serial dieter, went to her office holiday party she was hit with "dieter's" frustration - none of her frustration related to physical hunger or her body. Out of habit, my cousin's frustration around food was emotional and intellectual.

At first, Linda felt deprived about the party because she was trying to lose weight and would be surrounded by sweets. And then, she felt sorry for herself because she couldn't have what she wanted. She noticed her always very slender co-worker eating a chocolate brownie topped with a walnut in M&M-studded icing. Jealousy hit Linda like an empty fork.

Linda pulled herself together, as temptation rubbed like a cat with claws. Moderation was far from her mind. Just one bite would be the beginning of a binge. She was experiencing maximum, stressful frustration – trying to balance between self-discipline and self-indulgence and fearing a lack of self-control. Awful.

"Again and again, the impossible problem is solved when we see that the problem is only a tough decision waiting to be made."[1]

-- Robert H. Schuller

When frustration blocks the way, using patience, determination, dignity and prudence bring calm and relief. Using intuitive tools along with your senses puts you in control of eating choices. Things become less stressful.

You can have skills, equipment and experience but without the attitude of responding intuitively, you won't be able to balance emotion and reason. The decision to lean into and depend on your intuition, provides an entire, holistic warehouse of self-control artillery. Power.

Let's look at my cousin Linda's frustrations:

Feeling deprived to be attending a holiday party while you're on a diet frustration. Mentally and intellectually, it is clear that this is a party to celebrate the holiday with co-workers. It's an opportunity to network, spread good cheer, earn brownie points, and get insights into the personalities of co-workers. Emotionally, this frustration is the result of anger at herself and perhaps the sadness of nostalgia.

- **Tuning in intuitively:** Use foresight and see yourself walking into the room with your perfect body. This makes the important mind/body connection. Using your senses, feel self-respect, sense excitement in the room, see the delicious food, hear people talking. You see this party as an opportunity to socialize.

Feeling sorry for yourself because you can't eat what you want frustration. Emotionally, it is an expression of feeling disappointed in yourself, and a way of feeling unworthy and weak. You feel infantile. Mentally and intellectually, you may have some regret, but not much.

- **Tuning in intuitively:** Dignity does not bring the baby to the party. Use your eyes and curiosity and look back at the slim colleague with the amazing brownie, and notice: she's just holding it. You can see she's <u>not</u> eating it, but using it like a prop. This is a new perspective. Using patience, you have empathy for yourself and also some pride at the presence of your intuitive courage. Determination surges and you use prudence to enjoy yourself and to see how to use this situation to enhance your life.

Jealousy is a really unpleasant kind of frustration. Jealousy can only exist with feelings of being unworthy. This demeaning feeling is the product of inner dialogue built on a lot of hype. The hype feels like stress being whispered in your ear by a seemingly benevolent but really manipulative old uncle. When you are wallowing in a pit of self-disappointment and doubt, even an old fool seems wise.

- **Tuning in intuitively:** Using curiosity to connect with this jealous feeling, you recognize it feels demeaning. You connect with dignity, fight the hype and let go of being emotionally competitive. Choosing to feel worthy, you respect yourself with an open mind, tenacity and courage. This is self-discipline. Honoring yourself is putting up the good fight. You feel good about yourself, patience is your right hand and courage is your guide.

Frustration is a direct link to our survival instinct. When frustrated, you can have a victim mentality of feeling sorry for yourself or you can be determined to survive challenges of frustration with dignity. Fear of not having self-control over yourself around food is created by frustration. Turning fear into focus is the first act of every survivor.

Temptation

Temptation is the threat of giving up. Giving up brings on a deep sense of self-defeat. This is the opposite of the survival instinct.

- Experiencing temptation is an intuitive opportunity to prove yourself to yourself. It's the moment to be all that you can be.

- The way to focus is by using your senses with the intuitive tools to connect with common sense.

- Tuning into intuition keeps priorities straight.

"There is only one failure in life possible, and that is not to be true to the best one knows."[2] -- George Eliot

Binging

Binging signals a loss of self-control, the ultimate humility. Fear of binging and binging are not the same thing. While binging is self-defeat, fearing it is a heightened awareness that signals opportunity, Fear of binging is your 6th sense signaling a need to connect with your tools to stay in sync with yourself.

- By using intuitive tools for self defense - foresight, backed up by dignity, self-discipline and determination - you're covered. Instead of fear or frustration about the challenge of the situation, you feel strong about yourself and good about your choices.

- Your body feels a relaxed attitude of self-respect. Instead of eating the over-sweet brownie, you take a cue and carry around a napkin and 1/2 glass of soda.

- Because you see your ideal self-image clearly in your mind, there is no hesitation about how to handle yourself. Now that the office party is ending, you have made some new office connections and feel comfortable in your skin. Success.

Intuitively, frustration signals potential. Obstacles along the path to your ideal weight give you strength and energy to complete the journey. Frustration, anticipation, recognition, alertness and inner confidence are all intuitive. Learn to recognize frustration as a flag for new opportunity ahead. Then, push the doors open and forge your unique path.

> *"Nothing in the world can take the place of Persistence. Talent will not; nothing is more common than unsuccessful men with talent. Genius will not; unrewarded genius is almost a proverb. Education will not; the world is full of educated derelicts. Persistence and determination alone are omnipotent. The slogan 'Press On' has solved and always will solve the problems of the human race."[3]*
> Calvin Coolidge

Frustration is nature's way of ensuring survival:

A butterfly must beat its wings against the wall of a cocoon to break free. If someone tries to help by cutting a hole in the cocoon, the butterfly might be free from the cocoon, but its wings will not have gained the strength necessary to fly and the butterfly will die. In life there are always struggles - remember the butterfly. Be strong for yourself.

Intuitive eaters use curiosity to stay clear about what they're sensing, and dignity to honor their body. Ultimately, intuition leads to opportunities to live to the fullest. When you hit a wall of frustration:

- Have a flexible attitude by practicing patience and curiosity.

- Stay connected to what you sense by using foresight.

- Stretch to adjust to what is causing anxiety or frustration with the tool of tenacity. It will improve your ability to respond intuitively with patience.

Ways to avoid frustration include:

- Consider options (prudence). Take advantage of the opportunity to walk when it presents itself. Gentle movement is good for digestion and walking helps you stay limber. Also, activity diverts attention from what is frustrating so that you can regain your emotional equilibrium.

- Appreciating your friends nurtures your heart. When you realize that friends are a support system, it's easier to be true to yourself.

- Pleasant odors like cinnamon and peppermint make you more alert. Using lavender soap at night is said to create a more restful sleep.

- Use your sense of smell and discover its surprising impact on how much you eat. In general, the smell alone is the beginning of feeling satisfied.

- Take some time when you are in front of food. Pay close attention to what you see, taste, touch, and smell, noticing colors, scents and other sensory information. (curiosity) This decreases frustration, so you become calmer, and feel in control of your choices.

"You cannot have innovation unless you are willing and able to move through the unknown and go from curiosity to wonder."[4]
Markova

Eating alone is a good time to practice eating intuitively. Using the tools gives you the opportunity to practice the art of demolishing frustration. Connecting with your senses and intuition helps you realize that you are in control.

Everyone experiences frustration. Using tenacity, determination and courage as guides through frustration keeps us stronger and smarter than insecurity or ambivalence, and overrides old emotional habits. Repetition and practice using intuitive tools ultimately re-trains your brain. Intuitive eating becomes automatic and it's liberating.

Do the work.

- Use the tools as guides to recognize if hunger or frustration is driving your urge to eat. Then, make eating choices that make sense.

- Life is too rich and rewarding to pass by because it's hard. Every frustration is an opportunity to be true to yourself. It's not about the size of your effort; it's about doing it.

- Every action you take to be true to yourself is courageous. Don't underestimate who you are.

- Accepting frustration as an intuitive guidepost means you can recognize potential and create momentum in your life instead of seeing limits.

Frustration is good because it wakes us up. When the inner voice of intuition says we need to change something, it's usually attitude. Frustration, like eating, is deeply personal. Keep an open mind. When you change, everything and everyone in your environment changes how they relate to you. This is powerful.

Factoids:

> -Don't stand near the food at a buffet. Make the effort to stand somewhere else and you will eat less. (foresight)

-Walk around the mall twice before you start shopping. This is a great way to exercise your body while you exercise your shopping options. (prudence)

-During the holidays, eat before a party- have a hardboiled egg, an apple or an unsweetened thirst quencher. This takes the edge off hunger and makes it easier to avoid mindless eating. (tenacity)

-Remember to connect with your body and use all of your senses when you eat. Look at your food, touch it, smell it, chew and taste it. Enjoy eating and remember that you give yourself energy, build health and maintain your healthy weight by eating what feels and tastes good. (curiosity)

Am I Really Hungry?

Chapter 16 : Understanding Change

As children, we expect our bodies to change all of the time, so accept and deal with it naturally. In fact, right now your body is still evolving. Every cell is in a constant state of renewal. Every two weeks the skin is new; every five days the lining of your stomach is replaced; and your liver, which filters all of the poisons and drugs you consume, is new every year.

All of this regeneration requires nourishment. Different organs in our body have different nutritional needs. For this reason, it's natural for your appetite and food choices to vary.

"Variety's the spice of life; that gives it all its flavor."[1]
Wm. Cowper

When we don't recognize change, it's hard to deal with it effectively. Sometimes we see change coming, usually we don't. Using your 5 senses keeps you aware of changes in your body. Using the intuitive tools helps you cope with eating 'surprises'.

"Have patience with all things, But, first of all with yourself."[2]
St. Francis de Sales

Learning to eat intuitively is a change you control. Relying on intuition means achieving body goals while dealing with constant changes and challenges of life. Intuition does not desert you and is 100% focused on what's good for you. So enjoy the ride.

Often the challenge of change comes with frustration. Frustration is a signal that it's time to use patience to reconnect with clarity. Patience is the intuitive pause that automatically releases stress around changes because it resets your perspective. By relaxing pressure, patience renews your commitment to eating intuitively.

When you're clear and trust yourself, suddenly there are eating alternatives. Instead of reacting with tension or confusion, there is an arsenal of intuitive tools to depend on for guidance focused on achieving your goals.

"What we do willingly is easy."[3] William Shakespeare

All of the tools work together like a giant safety net. When you feel anxious about change, take a breath to pause and then tune into your 6th sense any way you can. Start where you're comfortable; remember that your 5 senses will keep you in tune with the present and to trust your instincts.

These intuitive signs of change are signals to use your tools:

Restlessness:

Restlessness is a head's up that comes as a nudge or ache. Often it's when you're considering a counter-intuitive decision, but before following through. For example, you're thinking about having a third slice of pizza or considering eating an entire box of cookies. As long as you're considering something, your memory is active and connecting with your intuitive voice. Uncomfortable heartburn memories and bloat memories stay in your mind. Foresight guides a restless feeling into calm.

Frustration:

Frustration means a situation needs to change or you'll feel defeated. It triggers the survival instinct. This impacts more than just what you're thinking, and a total connect with the arsenal of intuitive tools guides a release from the pressure of frustration.

'That Little Voice':

Use determination along with tenacity to separate that little voice from inner dialogue. That little voice is never destructive and always focused on what is best in the long term. So the next time you have a feeling that might be "that little voice," use the self-defense of foresight before listening to it. If the result is something that makes you feel good about yourself - it's intuition.

Anticipation:

Anticipation is an intuitive guidepost for navigating changes. It can feel uplifting or foreboding. With anticipation, use foresight for self-defense, and the inner-power of tenacity as guides to make decisions that honor your goals.

Gut feeling:

This sensation in the area of your belly feels odd or out of place. It means you're off-track. To understand where it's coming from and how to deal with it to your best advantage, start with curiosity.

First Impressions:

First impressions are intuitive when they are warnings from the senses such as: this smells spoiled, this tastes full of salt, that looks fattening, this feels rotten. But a first impression is not always right when speaking about food or eating. For example, it's foolish to respond to a first impression that tells you to eat an entire devils food cake with buttercream icing. Foresight and self-respect overrule the first impression in this situation. This is intuition in the form of common sense.

Intuitive Pause:

The intuitive pause is when you take a breath in and out and think about what you're about to eat. It is your way of using patience to check in with your body and intuitive tools to be sure you're clear about your choice. The pause is a sign of self-respect. One dieter I know put a sign on her refrigerator to remember to ask the question: "Pause... Y"

Sometimes when changes occur, intuition makes you 'pull back' which is a kind of 'pause'. This gives time to use prudence and dignity to navigate changes that impact your whole being. A pause is the opportunity to connect with the big picture. This brings a sense of control. A habit of doing the pause makes connecting with your tools automatic. You feel in sync with yourself.

Survival Instinct:

Our survival instinct is really a Live instinct! This means: be flexible, take chances by trying new foods, respond to longing in your heart, honor yourself and enjoy your senses. Be courageous and laugh often.

Habits

Dieting habits are like training wheels: they put you off balance and restrict your freedom. Changing from a mindset of dieting to intuitive eating is like going from riding a bike with training wheels to a two-wheeler. Training wheels give the habit of not being balanced, and they restrict biking freedom by slowing you down and making it clear that you are not capable of riding on your own. Give up training wheels by using courage and tenacity to ride on two wheels. Patience and self-discipline get you through bumps and bruises of experience and courage helps overcome fear of mastering two wheels. Ultimately, you find intuitive balance and become a free, easy rider.

- Observe yourself around food and your reactions to eating. Notice habits that trap you because they dictate when you eat, what you eat and how much you eat. When these habits are broken, new opportunities emerge. You'll find new taste treats and relate to your body differently. It feels wonderful.

- Habits create an attitude of entitlement. For example: since you have always eaten four slices of pizza, you expect it to be what you will eat. This ignores real hunger.

- Regular binging and stomach issues are the result of eating habits. Intuitive eaters look at each meal as the 'first time'. They don't always order the same thing because they first check in with the way their body feels.

- Using prudence keeps you about clear options your body needs Since clarity is a form of focus, and focus is a feeling of control, you feel strong and comfortable with new thoughts. The reward is knowing you're free to change your eating habits.

- Don't be critical of yourself. It's an old habit from dieting. Instead, be honest with yourself. Keeping clear about the truth is being intuitive; you stay deeply honest with yourself about what is real.

The bottom line is nobody needs eating habits. Eating choices should respond to physical hunger of the moment. It's relaxing to be spontaneous. Being relaxed gives you what you need to pause, be prudent and weigh the value of eating choices with personal goals. Life is good.

But if you sit down to eat with a rigid or tense attitude, you may not even taste the food or worse, be unsatisfied and end up binging later for comfort. Being relaxed connects you with eating to satisfy healthy hunger with dignity and enjoying the meal.

Counting calories or criticizing your choice is the opposite of being relaxed. Many people count calories out of habit. Calories are generic. Every eating experience, emotion and body is unique. Why not use dignity with prudence to enjoy eating what tastes good and let that be your guide? Trust your senses and use the tools to make it clear when you've had enough. Being relaxed with dignity puts you in control of your choices.

My cousin Linda has spent her life counting calories and chastising herself for enjoying cookies. Now, using intuitive tools, she's having fun and for the first time in memory, feeling good about her choices the next day. It's getting easier for her to relax, slowly but surely. Her history of being a yo-yo dieter has made relaxing slow going at first, but she's quickly seeing results and they're coming faster. Trust yourself and this process. It's a change to enjoy. Habits are like secondhand smoke - they sneak up on us. You, like Linda, can relax, trust your tools and enjoy eating.

This is what happened to Linda. She had a date for lunch and knew the restaurant had "bad" foods on the menu, so out of habit, she planned 3 days in advance to have a turkey sandwich. After lunch, because she did not feel satisfied, Linda came home and ate a box of cookies. The next day she experienced feelings of regret and low self-esteem.

I asked if she enjoyed the turkey sandwich, and this stopped Linda in her tracks. No, she didn't even remember eating it. Ouch. The intuitive commitment is to enjoy what you're eating or not eat it. Out of habit, Linda punished herself for three days before the lunch. The punishment was knowing for three days she could NOT have certain foods on the menu. Common sense made Linda resent this. In fact, she insulted her dignity by not respecting her self-discipline.

Of course Linda could have relaxed, met her friend for lunch, looked at the menu, listened to her body and mind and used her tools to have a meal she enjoyed. And it may have been the turkey sandwich. Surely a fresh turkey sandwich tastes much better than one that has been sitting in the corner of our mind for three days.

Habits from dieting are to restrain yourself, not trust your choices and ignore your body. Let go of feeling restricted and trust yourself when you experience change by depending on prudence and patience to be aware of options and of your ability to choose. Make smart choices using intuition; keep priorities straight and enjoy eating.

Eating intuitively is a pleasure. It's enjoyable to know you're being good to yourself and comforting knowing you're eating to stay feeling and looking good. It's exciting to know food will give you energy and it's rewarding to anticipate a delicious experience. Eating is a whole body, mind and soul experience. That's part of the enjoyment.

When the concept of relaxing at mealtime is hard, write down a list of reasons why you want to change and read it when habits are controlling your eating. This will help you get into the flow.

"You always pass failure on the way to success."[7] Mickey Rooney

Get in the flow of change by lightening up on yourself:

- Trying new foods and new eating habits is not easy. Use patience and courage. It's natural to be curious and healthy to feed your body variety.

- It's normal to feel a little frightened when letting go of old ways because emotionally, you don't know what will happen. It's habit to feel you'll lose control, but that doesn't happen because intuitive tools guide and protect you.

- Depend on intuitive tools. You will land strong.

- Often we get off to a false start and have to begin again. Old habits can be hard to let go of. The way to do it is with self-respect. Be kind and patience with yourself. Use natural determination and tenacity. Pay attention to your 5 senses to tune in and respond to the needs of your body. You're worth the effort.

Letting Go

Intuition is always an ally. It's your source of personal power to call on by using the tools when tension caused by eating challenges blocks the way. Recognizing change means responding to it. Using intuitive tools maintains momentum.

When you choose to be true to yourself it's natural to:

- Let go of the fear of being unable to change because in fact, you are in control of all eating choices and choosing to move forward in your life.

- Let go of frustration over gaining weight that made you uncomfortable and connect with the tools because you are committed to honoring your body and not torturing it or your emotional self. Your commitment is the anchor for healthy weight. Eating intuitively leads the way.

- Let go of the negative self-image of a person who yo-yos. Instead of listening to inner dialogue, remain in the present and respect your effort and commitment to change. Go with the flow. See and feed your ideal body. One meal at a time is a complete cycle for intuitive eating.

- Accept that you are who you are, and if you are true to who you are, you will remove pressure to be who you are not. By relaxing the vise-like grip of social pressure and self-pressure, you set yourself free.

"To err is human, to forgive Divine."[4] Alexander Pope

We resist natural change because we underestimate how powerful we are. Use tenacity along with determination and courage to follow your intuitive voice. You will be quietly impressed with what you achieve, because you are amazing.

Don't underestimate how much you know about yourself. Inner dialogue, which is created by years of conditioning, undercuts self-respect. Inner dialogue is like a callus. It can be rubbed off. You know your heart and your mind. Let them work with your senses to achieve your eating goal.

Emotional Eating

Emotional eating is a knee-jerk reaction that uses your body as its 'whipping boy'. It's self-abuse. Since emotional eating rarely has anything to do with hunger, it's a disconnect from your body. The emotional hot button is a bully easily set off by changes. Depend on tools of self-discipline and dignity to be honest about emotional behavior as you adjust to changes. It is never intuitive to compromise your inner dignity.

Instead of punishing yourself by binging when emotionally stressed, focus on the goal to connect with natural inner balance. Connect with your body, mind and emotions. Use patience and tenacity with dignity to experience a fresh opportunity to honor your body. Taking control of emotional eating means a regular commitment to dignity, patience and to being absolutely honest with yourself.

Our mind works with curiosity and patience to observe emotional 'hot spots'. Food is not a substitute for a best friend and will not ultimately raise your spirits. Emotional eating will create dis-stress instead of alleviating stress. When you face stressful changes, use foresight to plan a coping strategy that is not self-destructive. Constant changes regularly push emotional buttons. Intuitive eating tools relax the pressure of change.

- Watch for emotional hot spots that surround eating or food. Remember, with emotional eating, it's not what you're eating, it's what's eating you.

- Powerful emotions around eating are often misplaced and so, they are misleading. These become self-destructive because they distort priorities. Your mind, with the clarity of intuition, can recognize what is real and what is history, and how to respond positively to emotional stress.

Celebrate successes. Take joy in completing tasks and satisfaction in recognizing changes. Celebrating change by acknowledging yourself and your efforts, encourages momentum. Plus, it helps prevent depression and gives relief from stress related to eating.

Enjoy eating socially. Sharing mealtime slows down eating, nurtures the heart and stimulates the mind. All of this feels good and satisfies your appetites. It is a balancing act to practice having eating boundaries when eating with others. Foresight and tenacity are tools for comfortable socializing.

When possible, share the pleasure of eating when you're hungry. You'll discover that you eat less. Conversation is a good way to connect and since we can't chew and talk at the same time, it's helpful for pacing eating.

Becoming an intuitive eater includes changing your attitude around food and eating. As you socialize, share your new perspective about food. Everyone is interested in diet and eating. What you're doing is amazing and inspiring for others who feel trapped by diet dogma.

Appreciate

- Be thankful to have a satisfying meal. The fact that food is how we get energy to live is amazing when you reflect on it.

- Be glad if someone else cooked your meal. Notice how it looks.

- Appreciate the taste and smell. Chew well and you'll taste more and eat less.

- Enjoy the way your body feels as you treat yourself with respect. Enjoy the way you feel holistically.

- Remind yourself that you are satisfying your lifestyle goal of achieving a healthy, attractive body.

- Privately celebrate yourself and your intuitive tools.

Stay aware of how lucky you are to have choices about what you eat. On sitcoms, often someone jokes about finishing their plate because people are starving in China. In fact, people are starving all over the world. If you are reading this, then you are lucky.

Courage is a screwdriver in the intuitive toolbox. Sometimes you need to "screw your courage to the sticking place" to accept change in yourself and your patterns. Courage is bravery mixed with dignity. It takes courage to be honest with yourself. It takes courage to forgive yourself. This powerful tool opens opportunities to make decisions reflecting your priorities, and you feel good.

Courage unscrews the pressure of tension. Doing what is 'hard' to do can make you happier and ultimately makes life easier. Life is amazing.

Making changes in everyday aspects of life is an adventure because we don't know how it will turn out. Trusting your intuitive tools is a way of anticipating change. This is the comfort of listening to that little voice. Plan to succeed and you will absolutely learn about yourself and what you can do. You'll be impressed.

Humor

An important touchstone for going with the flow is having a sense of humor. Laughing at yourself is liberating and releases stress. By approaching eating challenges with humor, you are naturally more flexible. Being flexible keeps you open to possibility and opportunity.

Humor relaxes us and boosts our immunity. A recent study in Norway suggests that laughter can extend your life.[5]

Experience shows laughing at difficulties helps us think things through more clearly. Laughter is a humorous (intuitive) pause. Remember, the time you need to laugh is when you don't feel like laughing, because it changes everything by giving a different perspective. There will always be bumps on the road that jostle you off your path. Humor puts you back on track.

"If you want to make God laugh, tell God your plans." Folk Proverb

Everything changes. For ex: *"The latest research shows not every calorie is created equal, and different bodies use calories in different ways."*[6] *Psychology Today 2008*

Factoid:

The Cornell University Food and Brand Lab has a website that easily answers many questions about why, what, when and how much we eat. This practical site lists ways to shop smart, both in the supermarket and when ordering food, as well as practical tips for setting up your eating environment. Use curiosity and prudence, and check it out: **http://www.foodpsychology.cornell.edu/**

Am I Really Hungry?

Chapter 17 : **Create Your Plan**

"It's the possibility of having a dream come true that makes life interesting." Paulo Coehlo

An eating plan is a strategy for success. Every meal is a fork in the road of the journey of life and without a plan, we go in circles repeating self-defeating choices. There are cues and the point is to recognize them. Intuitive tools recognize and maintain inner balance, so eating when you're hungry and stopping when you're full becomes automatic.

Having a plan is a way of focusing. Focus is the magnifying glass in the intuitive tool chest that makes things stand out that you might otherwise gloss over. When you gloss over things, they haunt you. That haunting feeling is the 6th sense nudging to keep the momentum of this transformation happening.

Stay connected to a plan with direct access to your intuitive tools. This is how to do it. First, take a slow breath in and a slow breath out. This calming technique gives a pause to reconnect with your senses. It feels safe, like becoming more grounded. Now, remember this place of grounding. It is your 'safe place' where you can always access your intuition.

Second, because our mind responds to words, choose a word to be your trigger to connect with the 'safe place'. It has to just relate to you. Your trigger word should not be a name or have an emotional connection. Quietly saying the word is a private way to focus your intuitive connection. Importantly, you can use the word, pull this trigger and access your intuitive tools at any time.

Three very different trigger words are: "slim", or "dorje", or "pause". Tell yourself when you say "pause", you will be in a safe place. Combine pulling the trigger with a slow in and out breath. Practice pulling the trigger so at any time, you can calm and focus your mind. Plan to use it often and ultimately it will be automatic.

- Pull the trigger whenever you feel stress. A lot is going on and you want to stay clear.

- See the tools as self-defense. Use prudence and patience to pause, stop and connect with your senses to tune into your body.

Why have a plan if I'm listening to my intuition?

- A plan builds the foundation that creates and protects your chances for success. This built-in comfort zone becomes a fail-safe that keeps eating priorities clear. You maintain the connection with your body and identify details that relate to emotional and physical boundaries that impact eating choices.

- Having a plan gives you focus and focus keeps things ontrack. Incredibly, as you do this, you'll sense feelings of self-control and it's exciting. When you get excited about your plan, you're on a roll and when you're on a roll, it snowballs.

Eat with the purpose of nourishing yourself. The focus is to eat healthy, get energy and maintain a positive self-image.

- Purpose is achieved by observing physical needs with your senses and your mind.

- Observing is staying aware that needs are always changing. You respond to your body and environment and even let go of a plan when necessary.

- Goals are achieved by following through, which is best done in small gentle steps that follow logically and feel comfortable.

- Following through builds self-esteem that strengthens your intuitive connection.

- Always be open to a new mental map or strategy because "stuff happens". Being flexible is the tool of curiosity and using courage makes all things possible.

- When feeling uncertain, pull the trigger to go to the safe place where you'll relax and depend on the tools to connect with your intuitive compass. You'll find natural boundaries which guide and protect you.

You are master of your plan.

An intuitive strategy connects with the core strength of intuitive tools and your ability to be flexible. It reflects past endurance of emotional pain and lessons learned from your life experience. It's all about you.

When your plan is right, there is a moment of certainty. The plan is a unique ongoing process that affirms your body's constantly changing needs. It's a focus on best quality of life that doesn't change and this keeps your momentum forward. When in doubt around food, pull the trigger. It's safe to depend on intuitive tools to always keep on track.

Have a plan, follow the plan but don't fall in love with it. My experience is that the unexpected and the impossible do happen. Plans are dependent on circumstances beyond our control and there are times a plan doesn't work.

Hitting a bump in the road can become an emotional crisis. You may feel anger, disappointment, guilt or depression. Hitting a bump tempts us lose touch with dignity. Self-doubt opens us to inner dialogue instead of our inner voice. No matter what happens, intuition never deserts you.

Pull the trigger. Intuitive courage always has your back; you can sense it. Take a deep breath in and a deep breath out. You can depend on intuitive tools to pull through a crisis. Staying in the present, in fact, is a kind of momentum. Be kind to yourself. You are working hard.

Privacy and Boundaries

Privacy and personal boundaries are important and intuitive. They are essential to life as community. At the same time you're private, you interact with the rest of the world. By protecting your inner core you honor your body and in doing that, nourish your emotions and fortify your mind. When it comes to eating, plan to make choices that respect your privacy. You can always depend on the tools to maintain social, personal, emotional and physical boundaries in your daily eating routines. Trust your tools and yourself.

- Boundaries are the protective perspective that defines how to respect yourself. Boundaries are intuitive.

- Boundaries reaffirm self-control.

- Privacy is the safe place where you maintain your identity.

- Maintaining intuitive eating options is a private choice. Maintain your privacy.

General Plan Guidelines:

- Stop eating at the first twinge of filling. This gives you a chance to realize you're full before you overeat. It takes 15 minutes for messages to get from the stomach to the brain. Plan to give it time.

- Don't multi-task. When eating just eat, don't drive, walk, work or watch TV. When distracted you automatically may overeat, because you're not paying attention to eating or messages from your body.

- Pay attention to your food. Eat at a table and eat only what you want.

- Depend on intuitive tools to guide your food choices.

- Notice how you feel about yourself. When you feel in sync, you're using your intuition. It's as simple as that.

- Eat regular meals. Never let your body feel that it is starved. Feeling starved triggers a survival mechanism in your body to store fat and also can trigger a hormone that makes you want to overeat.

- Eat only when you are hungry. There is no other reason to eat - ever. It's common sense to listen to and respect your body.

- Walk more. In Europe and Asia where people are slimmer, walking a lot is common. If you feel too full to move after a meal, you overate. Walking aids digestion by helping things move inside you and also burns calories. Plus, walking is an excellent time to use all of your senses and pause to mentally check in with your safe place to reconnect with your intuitive tools.

When you create your plan, first be clear about connecting with your safe place; then use curiosity and dignity to:

- Experiment to determine the most satisfactory way to eat.
- Observe how you eat.
- Observe why you eat.
- Notice how you feel after the meal.

Build rules that you can live by into your plan.

- Stay clear about eating goals and enjoy the benefits of being in sync with yourself.
- Stop whatever else you are doing and observe yourself physically and emotionally, including stresses and needs.
- Think about what's in your best interest to fulfill your needs.
- Plan the easiest way to do what feels right.
- Act - Do it.
- Use your senses and smarts to make conscious eating a liberating habit.

Your goals will fall into place. Becoming an intuitive eater is very satisfying.

Staying On The Plan

Our mind is a trickster. It is where we rationalize and justify behavior. It's the place where we easily deceive ourselves. This has nothing to do with intelligence. It has to do with staying intuitively balanced.

For example: I had dinner last night at a popular food chain with K who is a PhD, an accomplished lawyer and educator, so we can say he's very intelligent. He's lost 20 pounds over the past two years and is committed to losing another 10. K mentioned that he has a lot more to accomplish in life and in order to do so, he needs to live a lot longer and has discovered that getting enough sleep, proper nutrition, and some form of exercise is his new diet. He practically glowed with happiness as he said this. He announced that in keeping with his diet, instead of ordering a fish fillet, he was going to eat "plants", meaning he was going to the generous salad bar.

K came back with a heaping salad smothered in a thick white salad dressing. I pointed out that the calorie count in the oozing dressing far exceeded what he would have had, if he had chosen to eat fish. K, embarrassed, agreed. He had deceived himself and ultimately, defeated his purpose. K "knew" the salad dressing was fattening, but ignored it.

The problem is K was emotionally driven with the salad dressing and not intuitively balanced. If he had used curiosity with patience to connect with his body and mind, K would have realized he was hungry for more than a salad. Or, maybe using the tools of dignity and prudence, he would never have heaped on the fattening dressing and instead, chosen to have enough dressing to flavor the salad but not drown it, or have the oil and vinegar dressing. He may have decided his body was asking for protein and ordered fish or a burger. We need to stay connected with our intuition and body and not be outwitted by inner dialogue. Trusting intuition keeps us balanced so we don't fall.

How do I know when I'm off plan?

If you're not in sync, you'll notice an edgy feeling, a nudge or even like 'something' is missing. Of course, your body lets you know right away when you're 'off-plan', but it's usually the mind or emotions that derail a plan.

These are the symptoms of being disconnected:

- **Denial** is when you ignore your intelligence. You disregard what you know from experience, which shows no self-respect.

- **Anger** is inner dialogue trying to out-shout common sense. Being angry, you berate yourself and ignore the obvious, which frustrates your being. This signals that you need an attitude adjustment.

- **Bargaining** is more inner dialogue trying to justify eating and is ignoring your goal. It's a battle of habit vs. insight. You need another perspective. It's time to 'pause'.

- **Depression** means insecurity wins; the emotional critical inner dialogue is victorious. This is a dark place that gives an illusion of being infinite. In reality, you can leave it with a flick of the switch, which is done by using your the trigger word.

- **Acceptance of uncomfortable choice** means you have disconnected from your intuition and followed the fork that is self-destructive.

Eating challenges are usually emotion-driven. Emotions can work for or against us. If we don't balance emotion with reason, we don't have a chance. Since diet and health are emotional hot spots, use curiosity and patience to see and know what you eat, as well as you see and know yourself. This way you can sort out what works and what doesn't work for your needs.

During an emotional crisis, your inner voice actively works to bring clarity, while inner dialogue tugs at your emotions with disconnected images, memories, hopes or fears. This is the time to connect with patience to pause, step back from the moment, pull the trigger and use determination, tenacity and courage to stay connected with your 6th sense. It's intuitive to seek balance.

When under stress, your intuitive voice becomes clearer, sharper and more commanding. This helps your body and mind relax and you find a refreshed perspective. Once you recognize inner dialogue and its attempts to manipulate you emotionally, you can ignore it. Use dignity to reject inner dialogue and find welcome relief.

Sometimes we feel uncomfortable because we cannot change an unpleasant environment or must eat new things or find ourselves around overly tempting foods. When you feel uncomfortable, use your trigger word to reconnect with your intuitive tools and get back on track. If you don't tune into your tools, you may fill up on bread rather than try something new or eat an entire plate of brownies because you are in emotional pain.

When your button is already pushed:

- Use your trigger word with a short in and out breath followed by two longer in and out breaths as an excellent way to reconnect with your body and your safe clear place. Then, connect with your senses and start fresh.

- Breathing in and out consciously connects your ears with your nose and chest, and this sparks with your 6th sense because breathing is directly connected to your survival instinct. Don't underestimate the power of your breath to bring calm.

- An immediate result is you re-focus your eyes, feel calmer and get a new perspective. Then it becomes natural to trust and go with your intuitive eating choice.

Panic

Emotion-driven confusion around eating is generally caused by doubt or fear, and when allowed to dominate, it connects with panic. Panic is never helpful. Panic is how emotions cop-out on us. It is the emotional way of giving up. When you notice panic, it's time to breathe, pause and regain the balance of your 6th sense. It's time to pull the trigger. The tool of dignity will put panic in its place. Dignity holds control by balancing your reactions.

Pain

As you endure emotional discomfort or pain, take a breath and enter your safe place. Decide with your mind and heart to use your intuitive magnifier: focus to look at options with self-empathy and clarity. Pain is a great teacher to the willing student and a cruel master to one who ignores it. Use your mind to pay attention to what is going on because something essential is happening.

The intuitive reaction to emotional pain is to protect yourself.

- Immediately go to your safe place to re-create your eating strategy.

- This re-establishes and reconnects with your boundaries. You can deal with this.

- Use your tools to recognize boundaries that protect and balance your emotions.

- Patience and perseverance clearly show there is always a way to achieve your eating goal. As you connect with your intuition, you start to relax because...

- You are in a comfort zone where you can trust yourself.

When we feel lost or emotionally stranded, it's common to revert to old eating patterns and habits. Being lost is not a location. When K drowned his salad with the white dressing, he lost his way; he lost his focus on his goal. The healthy habit of connecting with your safe place lets tenacity guide you to balance emotion with reason and automatically, you take the fork in the road that leads to feeling good.

Anger and Fear

Anger and fear are inflated emotional bullies. Sometimes the best way to punch a hole in the balloon of fear is to laugh at it. This brings it down to size. When fears are controlled, you relax and your senses open up. As a result, you're sharper, your mind is clearer and you find it easier to have a sense of humor. A sense of humor helps balance strong emotions because it gives a refreshed perspective and a pause.

Anger and fear are emotions that rob inner freedom by letting circumstances determine who you are. It is never intuitive to renounce your freedom or your dignity. By laughing at these bullies, you take away their power. Use humor to maintain emotional balance and let your tools guide from emotional turmoil or confusion to the comfort of clarity.

The physical plan is to honor, enjoy and empower your body.

- Eat only when you are hungry and only what you want. Intuitively, what you want is what you need. Eat what tastes "right". You know what feels good to your mind and body.

- Make it a point to use curiosity to understand the quality of what you put in your body.

- Your body is clearly a source of pleasure. It makes sense to feed it what feels good.

- Stay connected with your body by gently staying in touch with your five senses. Casually noticing what you see, hear, smell, taste and touch at mealtime becomes an easy habit. You'll discover that you intuitively "get" yourself and with little effort, eating becomes 'natural'.

- Never take hunger or your body for granted. Approach each meal as if this is your first meal. This keeps you in tune with messages from your senses and body.

According to Dr. Alan Hirsch, who is Neurological Director of the Smell & Taste Research Foundation in Chicago, *"if you pay attention to how food smells and tastes you will eat 22% less."*

Don't depend on a 'diet'.

- Recognize that eating needs are unique.

- Don't try to fit into an eating program or diet unless it feels good.

- Listen to your whole body and use your senses.

- Only do what feels right.

- Everyone has unique DNA causing our bodies to react quite differently to fats, carbohydrates, to types of exercise and to varied environments.

- We all think from our own perspective and each of us has a unique history. Your life is unique, your stress is unique, your needs are unique.

- Everyday things change, and that's why what you eat needs to be an honest response to what's going on in your life, who you are and what matters to you.

Depending on intuitive tools to stay clear about nurturing yourself through eating, automatically creates healthy boundaries. The intuitive eating plan is loose enough so that every meal can be modified based on what is happening in your life. The constant that never changes is depending on the 6th sense for guidance.

When we don't stick with the plan we experience stress, confusion, anxiety, hunger and emotional hurt. As you stay within the boundaries of your plan, there is a sense of harmony with your body, mind and emotions that produces healthy eating to maintain your weight.

The fact is, you can never depend on anyone but you to know what is truly best to put in your body. Self-respect, gratitude, humility, wonder, imagination and cold logical determination are guides, and for each of us they are unique. Intuition connects with the inner drive to eat well and live to your best advantage.

Be honest about what you experience. Personal integrity is the foundation of your plan and your intuitive compass.

- With stress caused by doubt or fear, use honesty to connect with dignity to applaud and support your choice to trust your intuition, and use patience to relax. You have made a commitment to really know yourself and to respect your body. This is good.

Depend on and trust your intuitive voice. Don't judge yourself. It's human to make mistakes. Recognize mistakes and let go of them. You will discover doing this frees you to move on.

- Success comes by acting on what you understand. Trust patience. You are evolving. Progress and change are naturally slow because growth is an organic process. The key to momentum is to keep depending on your tools for guidance.

- When it comes to what you eat: You are the person to answer to and you are in control of choices and have the answers to what you need.

- Ultimately, what makes this plan work is your commitment to follow through. Before you know it, recognizing and trusting your intuition becomes an automatic protective habit.

According to *The Flexitarian Diet* author, Dawn Jackson Blatner, RD, LDN[1], the biggest myth that people believe about weight loss is, *"If I exercise, I can eat whatever I want."* Ms.

Blatner, says that you should focus on food, not just exercise to lose weight. *"Exercise is for weight maintenance. Food control is for weight loss. 30 minutes of exercise every day helps to prevent disease, 60 minutes of exercise every day can help to stabilize your weight and 90 minutes of exercise every day is what is needed for weight loss."*

Factoid:

Brian Wansink, Phd. Director of Cornell University's Food and Brand Lab, has a great *"Mindless Eating"* quiz on his website. It is quick and fun to take and has lots of insights and suggestions that make sense. https://www.mindlessproducts.com/wp/wp-content/uploads/2009/09/mp_quiz.html

Chapter 18 : **The Mystery Tool**

Depending on your 6th sense creates new eating patterns and empowering habits. According to research, this creates new pathways in your brain.[1] Instead of banging your head against the wall to kill old habits, you're in sync with long-term priorities. This natural advantage is the result of using your intuition. The tool that makes it ultimately possible is Grace.

"Continuously stretching our selves will even help us lose weight, according to one study. Researchers who asked folks to do something different every day – listen to a new radio station, for instance- found that they lost and kept off weight. No one is sure why, but scientists speculate that getting out of routines makes us more aware in general."[2] MJ Ryan

Eating habits that feel like comfort zones can be ruts. Grace stretches beyond comfort zones to drive life priorities. A common eating habit is avoiding foods that are not familiar. This is being in a rut. Grace inspires courage, foresight, curiosity and prudence to connect with your inner appetite and guide eating to ensure best health. Grace is like crossing your fingers for good measure. It is when caring connects with courage.

21st century reality is we're busy multi-tasking with lots demanding attention. Distractions and responsibilities often result in impulsive or emotional eating. We're conditioned to see responsibilities outside ourselves as top priority. The way to deal with outside responsibilities to the best of your abilities is to keep your body healthy.

Fulfilling professional and social responsibilities is entirely dependent on our mental and physical health. Staying connected with intuition brings success and the energy to achieve it!

Intuitive eaters never forget that what they put in the body can empower or disrupt all aspects of their life. It's a fact that being good to yourself helps achieve your desired weight. It's up to you to make the best choices every day.

Weight Watchers identifies these self-defeating habits:

- Skipping meals, then overeating later to compensate

- Eating to cope with stress or other emotions

- Eating late, after dinner, during the night

- Binging- related to the menstrual cycle

- Eating nutritionally unbalanced meals

- Eating more when eating out

It makes sense to let go of useless habits and take control of your life. The commitment to use self-awareness to maintain a quality lifestyle is like peeling the layers of an onion to get to a flower. You peel by letting go of old habits to discover a new layer of self awareness and then another. Lifting off layers of vague awareness is a sweet experience. It's not always easy, but ultimately it feels good to be good to yourself. Grace is always present to remind you to try again.

"Knowing what you're good at and doing more of it creates excellence."[3] MJ Ryan

Grace

Grace a gentle intuitive kindness you experience as soft momentum, a nimbleness or agility that feels right. It is a heightened form of non-judgmental self-respect and appreciation that happens because you give yourself a chance to succeed. Grace always shines on your total potential and is always present intuitively.

Using grace increases awareness of what you sense, feel and think. It's a blind measure of all choices. Grace is having an open mind. It is giving yourself another chance whether you "think" you deserve it or not.

Grace connects caring and dignity with reflection and balance and this leads to intuitive insights. As you use grace, it appears to ease and encourage your way. Sometimes grace is when an idea occurs and sometimes grace is a door opening ahead because you're trying. For example:

- At a casual gathering you're handed a piece of irresistible flourless chocolate cake, the kind that melts in your mouth, with a small perfectly round ball of vanilla ice cream on the same plate.

- Emotionally and physically you want that cake. Dignity and self-discipline to make it easier to resist pigging out on the dessert. You have three choices, but only see two: (1). Cut the piece in half, giving the other 1/2 away or whatever it takes to get it off the plate or, (2) Eat the whole thing.

- You connect with your body and eat slowly, enjoying taste and texture. And it is really good. You use tenacity to stay focused on your goal, but ignore prudence and bite off too much, and now have indigestion. Prudence connects with your stomach ache, highlighting it to be remembered so as not to be exactly repeated, and then grace forgives, moving on to celebrate your experience of the cake with your eyes, nose, and mouth.

- Courage acknowledges the pleasure and congratulates your choice to eat intuitively by savoring the cake. This momentum is very exciting. Grace honors dignity driven choices and you feel good. You were in control, chose to enjoy 1 piece of this cake and are satisfied by your moderation. ·

There is a saying "Measure twice but cut once." Intuitive eaters depend on grace to observe life through a mindset of recognizing commitment and effort to make the right cut. Grace provides the perspective that is your edge.

Grace Always:

- Takes into account all aspects of who you are: mind, body and heart.

- Feels responsible in a loving way towards your being.

- Is considerate and protective.

- Is always there for you without being judgmental.

- Gives another chance to your senses, mind, heart and body with equal measure.

- Always acts as the stabilizer of your intuitive voice.

Empathy is understanding and sharing another's thoughts and feelings. Empathy with yourself is grace. To empathize with yourself, be aware of how you treat yourself. Be good to yourself.

Answer these questions with honesty and let your intuitive compass show how you self-empathize when sitting down to a big meal:

- Do I judge myself with Grace?

- Do I respect myself physically?

- Do I respond to my emotions?

- Do I trust myself to do the right thing?

- When it's time to eat, who am I feeding?

- Am I manipulated by inner dialogue?

- Do I forgive myself, and allow myself to move forward?

Empathy can be a group effort. If you are with a friend, it can be helpful to talk about what you observe about yourself, your tastes and needs, and learn how others cope with theirs. Part of seeing yourself can be learned through the eyes of others you trust. Part of seeing yourself can be learned by looking in the mirror.

Grace always connects with the 'Big' picture. It maintains a commanding perspective of our stress, efforts, flaws and beauty. Grace forgives and shows you are in control of what you choose to do.

> *"life is what we make it, always has been, always will be."*
> *Grandma Moses*

Use the pause of grace with your other tools to:

- Help understand how seeing a table full of desserts impacts your mind, body and heart, or to assess the impact of a broken heart and the value of a quart of ice cream.

- Understand yourself. As you stretch beyond habits to reach in with foresight to your reality and create the experience you desire, non-judgmental grace helps navigate the confusion and stress of going through changes.

Mirrors

Mirror, mirror on the wall... what are you really looking for? What do you see?

"Researchers have determined that mirrors can subtly affect human behavior, often in surprisingly positive ways. Subjects tested in a room with a mirror have been found to work harder, to be more helpful and to be less inclined to cheat ... Physical self-reflection, in other words, encourages philosophical self-reflection, a crash course in the Socratic notion that you cannot know or appreciate others until you know yourself."[4]   *NYTimes*

When looking in the mirror critically we see through a negative mindset. Women especially see their bodies out of proportion instead of the objective reflection. I saw a cartoon of a man and a woman looking at their reflections in mirrors. The woman had a healthy, slightly voluptuous, shape and saw herself as a pear. The man had a serious pot belly, and saw himself with broad shoulders and irresistible. We see what we're looking for.

The next time you look in the mirror give yourself a big smile. Remember you are seeing the person who wants you to have it all and is committed to eating well and feeling great. If possible look into your own eyes and laugh. It will change your perspective. If you must critique yourself, check out your posture. You look slimmer when you hold in your stomach and stand up straight. If you're not sure about your posture, stand with your back to a wall, if possible with your heels and your head touching the wall. Thrust your shoulders back to touch the wall. Now you're straight.

"Be patient with everyone, but above all with thyself. Do not be disheartened by your imperfections, but always rise up with fresh courage."[5] St. Francis de Sales

Don't be afraid of what you cannot do. Fear is one of those habits that are ruts. Use determination to turn fear into focus to achieve your goals. Only allow yourself to focus on the next correct action. Be gentle with yourself. Staying in the moment with foresight frees you from dwelling on what happened in the past and keeps the future open. life is big. Grace gives the ability to stay connected to the big picture. This feels good.

"How do you measure a year in a life?....In daylights, in sunsets, in cups of coffee. In inches, in miles, in laughter in strife....Measure in love."[6] Jonathan Larson, "Rent"

Old Habits

Old habits come from real places, and those places are history, which is the past. They include:

Physical causes:

- Chronic stress can mimic the chemical signals that feel like hunger. Fine tuning your intuition diffuses this because you learn to see it coming. Awareness puts you in control and alters old habits.

- Not listening to messages from your body leads to self-abuse. Caring about your body and recognizing that it is the source of energy you use to live allows new eating habits and choices.

Emotional causes:

- Sometimes you feel isolated, lonely, angry or lost and use food to connect with your world. Longing and frustration are both intuitive signals. Use grace with your tools, starting with curiosity and determination, and act with dignity to stretch to end these patterns and they will go away. When you follow your heart, you lose weight. Your intuition will always honor and protect you.

Inner dialogue:

- This habit sabotages time and again. Inner dialogue has no connection to your physical appetite. Often it is an unforgiving voice of resentment and negativity that holds you back. Use tenacity and dignity to identify and respond to your inner voice instead of inner dialogue. Once you connect with your intuitive voice, trust it. That little voice will <u>never</u> advise you to eat destructively.

Now that you're committed to being honest with yourself and to depending on your intuition to create the body and life you enjoy, you can let go of useless habits. Let a healthy body be the primary motivation for choosing food at every meal. Remember, it's healthy to vary your diet. This leaves room to enjoy a flexible eating lifestyle.

Grace helps you respect yourself, listen to and observe your body's signals and recognize when it's time for a change. Sometimes when you need to change, there is an intuitive nudge that feels like doubt. Grace guides you to relax and hear your intuitive voice. Follow where it pushes you. The reward is guaranteed.

Grace works to ease these challenges:

- **Discomfort** is when your pants are too tight, or energy level is off. When you don't feel good about yourself, eating is important for fixing it. Using curiosity to see if you are eating too many carbs, or not enough protein, or just don't feel nourished when you eat is part of caring. This means it's time to try different nourishing foods.

- **Stress** can drain energy or make you hyper. When stressed, the body reacts by tightening up, which means you need to eat gentler and be kinder with food. If stress makes it hard to find time to eat, use curiosity and prudence to help to get nourishment you need, and use foresight to stay healthy.

- **Self esteem** can be the result of falling in love or losing your job. Either way self-esteem is subject to being jerked around by destructive inner dialogue and by 'real life'. Tuning into your body and energy levels tells a lot. Self-discipline works with grace when you feel bad about yourself. Grace puts you back on track. Curiosity shows options because eating differently can be refreshing emotionally and physically. There is a thrill in the boldness of trying something new and a satisfaction in learning you liked the experience. Ultimately grace connects with courage to keep you on track.

- **Health** is intimately connected with our body. When you're rundown use curiosity to eat what you know is particularly nutritious. When you have a bug in your stomach, use prudence to just have liquids or to avoid heavy food. Grace keeps in tune with the whole picture of who you are: body, mind and spirit.

Confusion around eating happens when you're out of touch with your intuition. Impulsive behavior is the result. When you tune into your body and recognize your intuition, you won't be bullied by inner dialogue. Let patience and dignity guide your choices.

"Never be in a hurry. Do everything quietly and in a calm spirit. Do not lose your inner peace for anything whatsoever- even if your whole world seems upset."[7] *St. Frances de Sales*

Impulsive choices usually come back to haunt us. Grace nudges the tool of prudence to guide eating decisions with clarity of purpose. When we hurry, we miss things because we don't use our mind and we ignore our senses. Hurry leads to self-defeating choices.

Be Open To Possibilities

They say that the American Indians could not see Columbus's ships approaching the mainland until they landed because the Indians could not imagine giant white birds coming across the waters. The concept of sailing ships and another continent were out of their range of experience.

Visualize your dream body and your dream life. See yourself there. Like Columbus's ships- it may be right in front of you. Trust yourself and you will achieve intuitive goals. Let grace guide you to opportunity and the amazing.

Be Bold

Eating often presents the opportunity to try new foods. Anticipating what you will eat and predicting what something unknown will taste like puts you at a disadvantage. You don't know what you like before trying it. Let yourself out of the box of your experience. Be bold.

Now that you've decided to eat what's good for your body, it's time to make some educated choices. For example- I knew that beets were very healthy- for everything from preventing birth defects to preventing cancer. But, because I didn't like the way they looked, I never tasted them. But since I'm committed to eating to give myself every health and energy advantage, I ordered a goat cheese salad that included beets and mint because I like mint and goat cheese was protein I needed. Surprisingly the beets tasted sweet, and slowly over time, I learned to enjoy beets as part of my diet. Now, I love knowing the benefits I'm getting when I eat them. You never know what you'll discover.

"Seek and ye shall find..." is an expression that rings true. If you want to find food that's satisfying, tastes good, and leaves you feeling healthy – you will. That's a promise

According to the Rush University Medical Center: *Determining how much you should weigh is not a simple matter of looking at an insurance height-weight chart, but includes considering the amount of bone, muscle, and fat in your body's composition.*[8]

Maintaining Ideal Weight

People succeed without restrictive dieting to maintain an attractive, healthy weight by tuning into their bodies and depending on intuitive tools. They don't hold their body image next to a super skinny ideal. Importantly, by staying connected to the big picture, intuitive eaters believe good health and good eating deserve equal top priority and don't hold grudges against themselves when they 'slip'.

Grace is compassion that blends self-respect, dignity and patience with eating. When the truth is not easy, grace sees it as important and helpful. The process of facing the truth is continuous for each of us and as you move forward intuitively achieving your goals you'll discover facing the truth is like breathing, you can't stop doing it.

Apathy is a lack of enthusiasm. When being honest with yourself, be aware of apathy. It's a blah feeling that is slightly cold. Apathy is the absence of charity for yourself as well as others. Charity is part of grace; it's a new beginning. We all deserve grace for our efforts. When you stay aware by fine tuning your whole self, you are not apathetic. Forgive your past to let enthusiasm be part of the present.

Knowing yourself and using the tools grows into choices that liberate old self-defeating patterns. Grace is empowering. If you believe you are not honest with yourself about eating habits, try keeping a journal. But don't use it as a crutch to depend on. Instead, consider it a way to peel your onion and you'll know when you're done.

Grace is the fiber of your intuitive measuring tape. It is observing your changes from a place of dignity and patience. This quiet observation creates energy you can count on for an early, intuitive response.

You cannot be good to yourself without knowing yourself. Knowing yourself is to discover a sparkling gem. I'm not saying it's easy. I am saying it's worth the effort. Give yourself every chance.

Factoid:

Grace with yourself and with others is charming because it carries a big non-judgmental vibe. You have grace in your arsenal of tools. It's probably connecting with dignity right now. Use tenacity with determination to uncover your tool of grace and let it be 'back-up' whenever you're in an uncomfortable eating environment.

Chapter 19 : Falling Off The Wagon

"The best laid plans of men and mice often go awry."[1] Robert Burns

IT'S OKAY to fall off the wagon, but it's not okay to fall into a black hole.

My cousin Linda made a special dinner including homemade bread for her stepson and his wife. The next day she went to her job at a nursery school. There was a birthday party and they were serving her favorite cookies. Finding the cookies emotionally irresistible, Linda ate four and polished them off with a brownie. The emotional bookmark was comfort. This is falling off the wagon. So what? Life is full of surprises and throws curve balls with glee. It happens to everyone.

There are always exceptions to rules and circumstances that create different realities. Stuff happens and even great plans can fail. You recognize this intuitively by being curious. The important thing is to get back on the wagon and reconnect with perspective and grace. Intuitive eaters have a lifelong commitment to the process of trial and error, to forgiving themselves and then re-dedication. This is using patience and dignity.

"People don't come pre-assembled, but are glued together by life."[2]
Joseph Le Doux

Falling off the wagon is not about losing control. It's about hitting a bump in the road. There are no smooth rides in life. Everyone does things they later regret. Every person wishes they had made different choices. If we were all born perfect and knew how to do everything, when to do everything and what to do in all circumstances, then there would be no opportunity to grow. There would be no excitement. It's exciting to accomplish things. It is through accomplishments that you develop self-esteem. When a child is learning to color and he crayons outside the lines in the coloring book, it's part of the learning experience.

Sometimes the child who knows how to color inside the lines is tired, distracted, angry or joyous and he messes up. But on the next page the child starts fresh. He looks at the page, sees the outline for the art, picks up his crayons and colors inside the lines. We are all children, we're all always learning. We're always trying to do better, to please ourselves and not disappoint others.

When Linda fell off the wagon at the party she was responding to emotional bookmarks. The cookies, brownies and atmosphere were comforting. Eating more than made sense to her body brought Linda to another bookmark. Linda felt guilty.

Guilt is an emotion that occurs when we listen to inner dialogue instead of our inner voice. It happens when you believe you have disappointed yourself and to some extent others. Guilt is self-defeating when it makes you believe you've failed. From the perspective of failure, inner dialogue says you need to be punished. Then there is irrational anger towards yourself. With eating, the anger of guilt turns into self- abuse.

Had Linda listened to her inner voice she would have given herself grace and a chance to reflect about what occurred. This would have created a moment for Linda to reconnect with a sense of balance and feelings of control over her body and emotions. Physically feeling uncomfortable, Linda would have regretted her binge. With the help of patience and dignity she could make the choice to stop it. Instead, propelled by guilt, Linda responded to inner anger and punished herself.

That night Linda felt so badly about herself that she ate all of the leftover bread from the dinner party and the leftover cake. That's falling into a black hole. Linda was consumed with guilt and sadness and punished herself by abusive eating. Later that night she felt bloated, fat, bad, sad, stupid and full of regret.

Our risk/reward ratio in life doesn't come from reasoning. Instead it comes from emotional bookmarks. These are associations that emotionally connect current situations with similar experiences in the past. Emotional bookmarks are a way of using the present to repeat the past. They are associated with love, reward, punishment, guilt, self-worth, confidence, security, etc. Eating for "emotional comfort" because of guilt, loneliness, anger or shame, is self-abuse.

Self-abuse is a closed pattern of behavior. It is a way of being locked-up inside- mentally, emotionally and physically that needs to be dismantled. Self-abuse is insidious. It comes upon us gradually and is always hurtful.

You allow yourself to learn by using intuitive tools. This opens doors shut by closed patterns of behavior. You learn about yourself, what triggers you and why.

- Often smells make food seem irresistible. The sense of smell is located in our brain in the same place where emotions are born and where emotional memories are stored. Studies show that smell memories are strong and long lasting.[3] That's why smells of foods trigger emotional reactions. That's a physical reason why it's hard to resist emotional bookmarks.

Because intuition is always in the present, using the tools refreshes perspective to give a protective way to respond to bumps caused by emotional bookmarks. Intuitively you'll choose to get back on the wagon. Realizing that failure is easy, and willingness to try again, shows determination and being honest with yourself. Being true to yourself is using grace. Tenacity backed by courage is how to reconnect with dignity. Bravo!

By trying again, "what can be earned is a certain nobility- not in the sense of aristocratic status but in the sense of striving for quality and dignity of behavior in living."[4] Peter Leschak

Dignity confirms a fall off the wagon can be a learning experience releasing old self-defeating habits and an opportunity to change. An intuitive solution in a difficult situation doesn't allow self-abuse. When you observe choices with your senses, mind and heart and measure them with care it's obvious that you're in control to make a fresh choice that feels good.

Being true to yourself is maintaining control. It is paying attention to what you're eating and why. Because life is not predictable you intuitively adapt eating to fit needs and pressures. It is intuitive to have empathy for yourself, forgive bumps in the road and trust that you will achieve your goals.

Everyone falls off the wagon. We live in a pressurized world that promotes gluttony and selfishness. Advertisement and commercials urge us to gratify every craving and experience every taste sensation, but at the same time to never get fat. That is not possible and when overwhelmed by pressure outside of ourself, we lose touch with common sense.

Instead of responding to needs and respecting our physicality, we strive to look like models whose image is often airbrushed and not real. Having a distorted body image and a misplaced relationship with yourself is an intuitive disconnect. For many who ride the tide of dieting, food is seen as reward, compensation or even a weapon.

For intuitive eaters food is a tasty way of fortifying daily life. But for many, food is an obsession. Obsessing can be a way of avoiding. If you're obsessed with food then you need to ask yourself, why? Perhaps thinking about food is a way to avoid thinking about other things? When I'm depressed or frustrated I will often play solitaire on my computer.

Letting myself obsess with the game gives me a false sense of being free from the discomfort of what's bothering me. Of course since it's not true, it's not healthy and what I'm avoiding doesn't go away. Still, I allow myself a ½ hour of indulgence and then very consciously restrict myself because I know in my mind that life just isn't that dark. I am able to do this by consciously going to my safe place and using my intuitive tools, which wakes me up to the fact that I'm sitting in a holding pattern. Then, with prudence, determination and grace, I remember my commitment to myself to live the best life possible.

Doing this requires that I examine myself honestly and face the truth about my behavior. To fine tune and stay on track is lifelong work of trial, error, forgiveness and re-dedication. It means being honest with yourself again and again. It's hard, but the reward is an immediate reconnect with dignity, which feels great.

When you're off-track the way to face the truth is:

- Observe your behavior with courage, curiosity, dignity and patience.

- Acknowledge errors with self-discipline, determination and kindness.

- Forgive yourself with grace.

- Rededicate to doing what's right for you with courage, foresight and dignity.

This is what my cousin Linda did after her day and night of binging. She examined how she felt physically and emotionally. Looking at herself honestly, Linda realized that spiraling down the black hole was increasing the damaging emotional feelings of self-loathing and that she wanted to stop it. She decided to forgive herself and rededicate to healthy eating. Forgiving allowed Linda to feel deserved self-worth, and to resume eating intuitively the next day.

One day at a time is all you can ask of yourself. *"...experiments in truth require commitment, attention, and patience. We have to decide to settle for nothing less than the best life; we have to be awake to how and why we do things and what sort of people we are becoming. ... The crucial thing is to discover the habits that kill our souls and those that nurture them."[5]* John Loudon

Being true to yourself is liberating. Trust your tools to guide your choices. Limit how much time you think about food. There are other important things in your life. You eat three meals a day which means possibly a minimum of three hours a day to think about food. Try to realize that more than this is dishonest because it is using food to avoid living your life. Ouch.

6th sense eating creates and recycles feelings of abundance. This includes a gratitude for life's gifts of strength of mind and physical well-being. You get this by eating with attention and appreciation exactly what you want. The secret of success is knowing when you're satisfied by staying aware of your senses and signals from your body.

Factoids:

A goal of eating intuitively is to enjoy foods that fill you up with nourishment to provide hours to be productive and enjoy your life. Here are some foods that fill you up:

- Eggs: These are a great source of hunger-satisfying protein (about 6 g per egg). A recent study found that women following a low-fat diet who ate 2 eggs for breakfast at least 5 days a week lost 65% more weight and averaged an 83% greater reduction in waist circumference.6

- Almonds: These tasty nuts contain the healthy monounsaturated fatty acids, good-for-you fats that keep your appetite sated for hours. Studies back this up—one found that after 6 months, dieters whose eating plan included plain raw almonds lost 63% more weight, lost 50% more body fat, and shrunk their waistlines 55% more than those on a high-carb diet.6 The maximum number to eat at one time is 20.

- Avocados: A few slices with a little lime juice is rich, satisfying, and loaded with important nutrients, including those healthy monounsaturated fats, plus vitamins and minerals like potassium and folate. They are not calorie free, but a few slices have between 50 and 75 calories and will make any salad or sandwich much more satisfying.6

- Apples: One study found people who ate one apple before every meal lost 40% more weight than those who didn't. Plus, they're low in calories—about 65 for one that's medium-size.[6] I prefer to eat apples sliced like a finger food.

- Oatmeal: This contains high amounts of soluble fiber, which slows digestion and keeps us full for hours. A study found that people who ate plain oatmeal for breakfast every day and also walked an average of 15 to 30 minutes daily lost about 10 pounds in 12 weeks.[6]

- Peanut butter: Despite the name, peanuts are actually a legume (plant) not a nut, but they're still high in craving-quashing monounsaturated fats, and research has found that dieters who snack on peanuts or peanut butter lose more weight than those who don't. Read the label before you buy because popular brands are loaded with salt and sugar. Buy organic or natural peanut butter that does not contain sugar and salt. Spread some on those apple slices next time you get the 4 pm munchies.[6] Limit your munchie intake to 2 tablespoons.

An article about decorating called: **Weight Loss by Design**[7], made me curious. This is what I learned:

- Furniture is important for healthy eating because when we eat standing, or on the go we are "more likely to shovel in more calories" than we need. They suggest eating at a table sitting on a chair, not watching television, but instead, noticing what we're doing. As an intuitive eater, also be sure to enjoy your meal.

- Place settings manipulate us. If we eat meals on plates that are 9" across instead of 12" and choose bowls that hold 17oz instead of 32oz for soup or dessert we'll dish out less food, "which may, in time, translate to smaller jeans size for you."

- Lighting affects how fast we eat. According to Dr. Brian Wansink, director of Cornell University's Food and Brand Lab, very bright lights make us eat faster and very dim lights encourage us to be less inhibited and eat more desserts. Moderation always works best. ;-)

- Color of the walls, according to Dr. Wansink also impacts how we eat: Red and orange make the environment stimulating, so we rush; and blue and green encourage us to linger, and so succumb to temptation to overindulge. He recommends neutral shades like white, grey, or beige.

Using our senses reminds that it's important to balance internal messages with our external environment. It is always good to use curiosity to learn because in fact, you don't have to re-paint your walls or buy new furniture but you do need to know your options.

Knowing options helps you make wise choices. Protecting yourself is knowing when you are being manipulated by plate size or lighting or emotional bookmarks.

If you're thinking about re-decorating or making other changes, use prudence to weigh suggestions from others before assuming they are right for you.

Am I Really Hungry?

Chapter 20 : **Stress**

In our fast paced world so much is happening it's not surprising that we don't remember if we remembered to eat lunch, or even what we ate. We're stressed; we feel conflicted. Quite possibly we're getting messages from that little voice and inner dialogue non-stop at the same time; so we tune both out.

Stress hits us emotionally and our reaction is physical. We get nervous or freeze, overeat, obsess or lose our appetite altogether. Stress creates situations where we lose perspective until we remember to connect with our inner guidance system because common sense is an emotional anchor that pulls in the big picture and defuses stress.

Everybody talks about stress. It's an intuitive disconnect that knocks us off balance. Stress is part of life and you can control how you react to it by using your intuition. It is just another bump along the road. You can deal with it

The most powerful thing to do when stressed is use your senses and your tools to refresh your perspective. People have their own ways of defeating stress. Britney Spears reads:

"Every night, I have to read a book, so that my mind will stop thinking about things that I stress about."[1] Britney Spears

Reading takes Britney's stress energy away from her emotions, which takes away its power and this ultimately restores her emotional balance. Reading a book gives Britney a connection with her logical thinking mind and makes that voice louder then emotionally manipulating inner dialogue. She reconnects with intuition by connecting with her mind. Her survival instinct is to take a pause from inner dialogue and gain a fresh perspective.

Distracting stress by exercising your mind is a way of regaining perspective. This way of exercising your mind is good for reducing stress; it is how you 'feed' your mind.

Prolonged stress creates imbalances with the immune system, encourages hypertension, heart disease, sleep disorders and more. Did I mention overeating? Diets are, by definition, restrictive.

Feeling restricted creates stress which can create weight gain and prevent weight loss.

When stressed you may be distracted, not think clearly and vulnerable to being seduced by food. You might use eating to avoid thinking about what's stressing you or may obsess over food and gorge without mercy. When stressed, people eat mindlessly, often using eating as a release valve. Ouch.

Because stress impacts hormones, we respond to it physically and because it turns up the volume on inner dialogue we are emotionally manipulated. Stress feels really serious because stress takes itself very seriously. You may "need" to eat the entire box of cookies and the ½ gallon of ice cream when you're stressed. With practice, using intuitive tools creates a protective boundary between what's stressing you and what's best for you.

Possibility and Opportunity

Intuition keeps in touch with possibility and opportunity so you're aware of the 'big' picture. Common sense drives you to live your best life. It's intuitive to go to your safe place for grace when you're stressed.

Connecting with intuition is how to ground yourself and maintain a healthy perspective. With dignity and patience you make eating choices that respond to your body and not your stress. An open perspective means you have more options.

Laughing is a stress buster. Having a good laugh every day is like eating an apple a day. It keeps the doctor away. Studies show that laughter activates our most protective immune system cells, increases blood and oxygen flow through our body and manipulates hormones! Think of laughter as an organic mega-vitamin pill.

"Studies show that the physical act of smiling can signal your brain to halt the negative, mood-altering effects of stress."[2]
Roz Trieber, educator, author, HumorFusion.com

They say, 'laughter is the shortest distance between two people.' In fact, humor equalizes tension creating emotional balance and releasing stress. According to Reverend Laura Gentry, also known as 'Laughing Laura'[10], "Laughing makes the heart connect. It makes small issues dissolve and enhances our ability to forgive."

Laughing gives a refreshed perspective. It's an opening for the pause that refreshes. Sometimes while using intuition to follow thoughts with dignity and determination and finding patience in your tool chest, you might discover humor. You may experience it physically as a laugh. When you do the intuitive pause and recognize the bully of stress, you regain perspective. Life can be funny.

Connecting with intuition relaxes your mind so you perceive what is real, differently. When you perceive reality from a fresh place your physical reaction is different. An open mind diffuses stress. There is a saying, "If you all throw your problems in a pile and see everyone else's, you'd grab yours back."

Intuitive eating gives energy and self esteem and in general you're okay when you're being true to yourself. You're learning all the time. But even though staying connected with intuition is a stress buster, it doesn't stop stress from coming. For example, even when using curiosity and prudence to shop wisely for food, it's not easy.

"That's why you should be wary of hot-button words on food labels. "Reduced-fat" products usually have less fat and "all-natural" foods often do come from ingredients actually found in nature. But not all health-related words on food packaging are defined by the Food and Drug Administration, leaving certain gray areas for manufacturers to exploit. So while those phrases, and others like them, would seem to indicate that the products inside the packages are somehow "healthy," the reality is often something very different. As likely as not, "reduced fat" means "increased sugar."

" As for products that are "all natural"? Well, so are hurricanes and tidal waves. And the most deceptive word of all? That might be the word "healthy." Because there is no way to really define it, the FDA has no way to regulate it. And just about anything out there can be healthy—or unhealthy—in the right amounts. In this slideshow, we dig deep, below the surface labels, and expose the real truth behind some of the food industry's most specious health claims." EAT THIS NOT THAT, Men's Health Magazine,

A hormone called ghrelin is activated by chronic stress.[4] Our body interprets stress as hunger because ghrelin tells the brain that we're hungry. This hormone's official job is to decrease depression and anxiety, but according to Dr. Jeffrey Zinman, of the University of Texas Southwestern Medical Center, *"An unfortunate side-effect is increased food intake and body weight."* His associate Michael Lutter said, *"Our findings support the idea that these hunger hormones don't do just one thing. Rather, they co-ordinate an entire behavioral response to stress and probably affect mood, stress and energy levels."*

This means that stress you may experience at the expense of putting a child through college can be affecting your metabolism. Stress affects you holistically. Intuitive eating helps deflect stress because it's eating from a holistic perspective.

The Holy Trinity of beating stress:

Be honest with yourself.

Connect with your senses.

Use the intuitive tools.

A trinity is 3 powerful things existing in a co-dependent relationship. In the intuitive trinity, Mind, Body and Soul equally support the other, which keeps us whole. When we experience stress, the trinity shatters. We feel splintered. Ouch.

Some ways to diffuse stress:

- Quick nap – 20-30 minutes
- 10-20 min exercise like walking

    -Enhances mental state

    -Reduces risk of heart disease,

    -Improves blood pressure and sugar levels

    -Boosts metabolism

- Listen to music for 15 minutes.

    -Studies at the Cornell Center for Complementary and Integrative medicine, state this can lower stress hormone levels by 25%.

- Breathe and count.

    -Breathe out for twice as long as you breathe in.

    -Breathe in and count to 8. Breathe out and count to 16.

-Repeat 3 times. You will feel like a different person.

Natural childbirth is certainly stressful. I discovered that the Lamaze breathing technique for labor pain works for all stress. The quick short repeated out-breath from the mouth works. Instead of eating late at night stuffing stress inside, blow it out in the privacy of your kitchen and have a good laugh.

Feeling clean intuitively feels good. Pampering your body with a relaxing bath or shower diffuses stress. Pampering is the measuring tape of kindness that validates and re-affirms an emotional balance with your body. It focuses on your body as a source of pleasure and relays information about how your body feels to your mind, which is an intuitive connect.

Stress creates an illusion of being alone. Eating dinner with friends or family is a easy way of connecting. Sharing concerns puts them in perspective. Sometimes just hearing someone else vent about their stress makes you realize you're lucky or having someone to share problems with gives a perspective that opens your mind. Noticing when you can be grateful helps balance stress.

"Gratitude unlocks the fullness of life. It turns what we have into enough, and more. It turns denial into acceptance, chaos to order, confusion to clarity. It can turn a meal into a feast, a house into a home, a stranger into a friend. Gratitude makes sense of our past, brings peace for today, and creates a vision for tomorrow."[5]
Melody Beattie

The more you use curiosity and choose to be flexible, the more you notice the bigger picture. This helps make eating choices that give a good quality of life. Connecting with curiosity and foresight leads you to look around the corner and see what's real. Often what we're told is more, is really less.

When going through a stressful period, do the intuitive pause by asking yourself a series of questions. After each question, I have put one of the tools that will help you to re-gain your intuitive connection with balance. Pull the trigger and be honest with yourself.

Use your senses and intuitive tools together to answer these questions:

- Am I clear? - Curiosity
- Am I wise? - Foresight
- Am I tough? - Tenacity
- Am I strong? - Patience
- Am kind to myself? – Grace
- Do I relax? - Dignity

If you're curious about how you're doing 'intuitively', rate your answers on a scale of 1 to 4. The lower your total number the better the score:

(1) You are using your tools.

(2) Sometime you use the tools.

(3) You're unsure.

(4) You're confused.

Observing with your senses and mind connects with your intuitive voice and helps to navigate the zig-zag path of life. Because stress is a fact of life, it feels best to stay clear about changes. That's how to let go of what was and stay connected with what is.

Five elements you can count on to stay connected with your truth are:

- Dignity - of self mastery
- Humility - clarity of perspective
- Heart – your feelings
- Spirit – your intuitive voice
- Tenacity - commitment to yourself

Being honest with yourself renews an intuitive lifestyle that diffuses stress.

Disconnected eating habits can make you a medical statistic. Medical bills that result from not feeding yourself with intuitive tools are avoidable stress. A clear intuitive goal is to eat for mental, physical and emotional health at every meal. Use your senses with curiosity to eat what will nourish and energize you.

"According to the Centers for Disease Control and Prevention[6], three-quarters of health care spending now goes to treat "preventable chronic diseases." Not all of these diseases are linked to diet — there's smoking, for instance — but many, if not most, of them are.

We're spending $147 billion to treat obesity, $116 billion to treat diabetes, and hundreds of billions more to treat cardiovascular disease and the many types of cancer that have been linked to the so-called Western diet. One recent study estimated that 30 percent of the increase in health care spending over the past 20 years could be attributed to the soaring rate of obesity, a condition that now accounts for nearly a tenth of all spending on health care.[7]

The American way of eating has become the elephant in the room in the debate over health care." Michael Pollan[8]

Peace of mind is the opposite of feeling stressed and comes from taking care of yourself. It brings a nurturing attitude so when shopping for food or eating, you have an open mind. Get creative with what you eat.

Breaking patterns creates a refreshed perspective and reduces stress.

- Try new fruits or vegetables.
- Eat dinner for breakfast and breakfast for dinner.
- Eat foods from other cultures: Chinese, Italian, Mexican, Indian, Japanese, French, etc.
- Skip a meal.
- Cook something original.
- Give yourself the task of enjoying what you eat.

Because intuition connects with a sense of order in our lives, time management is another intuitive stress buster. Order brings awareness of balance and harmony as you diffuse stress. Being fine-tuned is being on top of your game. That's when you feel least stressed. Give yourself time to enjoy your meals.

Make the choice to:

- Stay connected to your safe place and use it to protect and defend your life.

- Pay attention to food when eating, notice if it's satisfying and healthy.

- Take time to relax and reconnect with common sense and your body by using your senses as you go through the day.

When you notice the stress in your body, you can release it in healthy ways.

Some easy suggestions:

- Get at least 30 minutes of moderate exercise by being aware of your posture whenever you walk - hold your head high and your shoulders down and back. Look at where you are going. Smile more.

- When you are sitting - hold your chin up, bend your elbows and slowly flap your arms like a bird. Bend and straighten your legs. Rotate your feet several times in both directions and feel the stretch in you ankles. You can do this any time.

- Stretch out your arms and rotate your hands forward 3 times and backwards 3 times. Do it a few times and notice how good you feel.

- Do something fun.

- Do anything that will put a smile on your face- this includes looking at photos of loved ones or watching a sitcom on TV.

- Being happy, excited or content lowers levels of stress hormones that are linked to heart disease. Enjoy little things, be happy.

"When the heart is at ease, the body is healthy." Chinese Proverb

Stress can create feelings of losing control that make us feel hopeless. The way to get back on track is to ask: What do I really want? And then remind yourself that the choice is yours. You own it.

Being honest with yourself releases stress and is surprisingly gratifying. What are you waiting for? Every year you pass the anniversary of your own death. Live fully now by creating a rich healthy eating lifestyle.

When you begin to sense stress, use grace with kindness to re-commit to being honest with yourself.

The 12-Step Program

A 12-step Program is a set of guidelines outlining a course of action for recovery from addictive or dysfunctional behavior. The pressures of stress can create this behavior without us realizing it.

The IntuEating 12-Step Program to alleviate stress:

1. Admit stress impacts your eating.

2. Realize however good or bad a situation is, it will change. Use your senses and mind to analyze the environment and place yourself away from the food table.

3. No one is in charge of your happiness but you. Make peace with your past so it won't screw up the present. You know what you're doing.

4. Take a deep breath in and then exhale all the way to connect breathing with your mind and body. Pull the trigger and go to your safe place inside to renew your intuitive connection. Trust yourself.

5. Connect with a strategy to diffuse stress and create a new perspective- let your mind and body distract you from the emotional bully of stress. Read, exercise, or find someone to talk to - create a strategy based on your ways to feel good about yourself when you are in a stressful food environment. Use foresight.

6. Have patience with yourself - just take the next small step with tenacity focused on your goals. Depend on your tools to maintain inner balance.

7. Remember, by honoring your whole self you won't regret this in the morning.

8. Maintain the comfort of balance by checking in with your secret place and using your tools, especially dignity and patience. Reconnect with the image of your perfect healthy body.

9. Be aware of your 5 senses to stay connected with your 6th sense.

10. Tell a joke, listen to music, take a walk or exercise to distract and diffuse stress.

11. Recognize your mindset is empowering and let it work for you. Remember your trigger word and use it often.

12. Stress comes and stress goes. You are in control of your eating choices. Choose to feel good.

Factoids:

- Peppermint leaves have been used to ease headaches and aid digestion for more than 2,000 years. Peppermint oil is a key ingredient in many decongestants and in remedies for irritable bowel syndrome. Consider drinking peppermint tea instead of coffee after a big meal.

- Parsley is a natural diuretic and can ease pre-menstrual bloat. It also has high vitamin C content. Chewing parsley after eating a meal heavy with garlic, freshens your breath. The next time it's on your plate decorating your fish, chicken or potatoes, try it.

There are many tips on the Internet for beating stress. Woman's Health lists nine foods "that will keep you calm" at **womenshealthmag.com/files/best-tips/beat-stress.html**

- Almonds – about ¼ cup contains vitamins and anti-oxidants that boost our immune system.

- Pistachios – about a handful helps to lower stressed out blood pressure according to a 2007 Penn State study.

- Walnuts – about ¼ cup is good for the heart anytime.

- Avocados – ½ of one is very high in potassium, which reduces blood pressure according to the National Heart, Lung, and Blood Institute.

- Skim milk – up to four or more servings a day provides calcium that can reduce muscle spasms and soothe tension.

- Oatmeal – unsweetened, according to Judith Wurtman, PhD., co-author of The Serotonin Power Diet, the slow steady digestion of carbs in the form of oatmeal creates a smooth steady flow of the relaxing brain chemical, serotonin. Also regular unprocessed oatmeal tends to keep us feeling full for hours.

- Oranges – high in vitamin C, plus a naturally sweet energy boost

- Salmon – a three-ounce serving is full of omega 3 fatty acids, which according to the Journal of the American Medical Association, protects against heart disease.

- Spinach – one cup provides magnesium that lowers stress levels as well as protecting our heart and our brain from stress related illness. It has one of the world's healthiest food ratings.

- Popeye made himself super-strong by eating spinach, "he may also have been protecting himself against osteoporosis, heart disease, colon cancer, arthritis, and other diseases at the same time."[9]

"Give your stress wings and let it fly away." Terri Guillemets[11]

Am I Really Hungry?

Chapter 21 : Bondage

Intuition is a natural bond between your senses, mind and heart. It is a connector that keeps channels open. Bonds make sense when we're aware of them. You have healthy bonds with friends, family, responsibilities and pleasures in your life. These create a sense of control and stability that feels like balance. Any healthy bond is a strong intuitive connection.

"A bond is necessary to complete our being, only we must be careful that the bond does not become bondage."[1] Mrs. Anna Brownell Jameson

In the popular science fiction movie, The Matrix (1999), what people experience as real life is really a simulated reality created by aliens to pacify and subdue humans while their bodies are being used as fuel. People are in a dream world that feels familiar and comfortable. It is as if they are living while, in fact, life is literally being drained from their bodies. The worse form of bondage is when we don't realize we're enslaved. When habits become involuntary servitude, you're in bondage.

Cultivated habits and unconscious habits create bondage. Intuitively, this feels uncomfortable or wrong. When habits make you feel bad, use curiosity with determination to notice what you're doing to cause this feeling. Curiosity helps you be flexible to protect your needs, while determination renews a commitment to enjoying life and grace gives the cushion of a non-judgmental perspective on what you're doing. Bondage is a weak link. It's weak because it's a disconnect from your intuition.

Bondage : The state of being bound; condition of being under restraint; restraint of personal liberty by compulsion; involuntary servitude; slavery; captivity; obligation.[2]

Slave to The Scale

When something you do manipulates your emotions so you become dependent on it for self-validation - this is bondage. You're in the matrix. The bathroom scale has become a way people judge their self worth. When you decide you can have dessert today because of what it says on a scale, you have lost connection with your body. You're treating yourself from the neck down as a piece of meat to be weighed - Not a very attractive image.

Emotionally. the scale turns us into slaves. It is the silent taskmaster that shows us what we are worth. NOT!!! In fact, a scale does not provide validation of your efforts. Weight management is not scale-dependent. Many intuitive eaters don't own scales. If they do use one, it's a form of measurement as a response to curiosity, but not a way of self-validation.

The scale is not your friend. My landlady's scale has an annoying, judgmental and ultimately absurd function: every time she steps on it she hears how much she weighs compared to the last time! She says it's unpleasant, demeaning and personally invasive. The last time we spoke, she was trying to find a way to turn it off. Her scale actually reaffirms hostile and demeaning inner dialogue. Ouch!

Scales are rigid. Right here, a light should go off. Life is not rigid. In fact, it's the opposite. Life is full of surprises and not consistent from day to day except for the fact that the sun rises and sets. What happens in between is a matter of circumstance, timing, luck, convenience, focus and responsibilities. None of this is rigid and all is real. Judging yourself by numbers on a scale is misleading. Judging yourself at all is not intuitive. Observing yourself with patience and dignity and being tenacious is how to weigh yourself intuitively.

At all times we're tossed about on a sea of circumstance. Hormones are always in flux. Thoughts are constantly being streamlined to fit in the molds of life formed by responsibilities. You experience physical stress caused by exercise, both intentional such as working out, or not, such as lifting groceries, carrying children, racing to a meeting or driving in bad traffic. Everything impacts nutritional needs.

It's intuitive to want a stable weight that reflects your goal for looking and feeling your best. In fact, body weight is naturally in a state of gentle flux. For women, it can vary as much as 10 pounds a month with their period. For the rest, a variation of three to five pounds at any given time is natural. For some, weight is always the same; others easily carry water weight. We are each holistically unique.

No one loses weight at the same rate or the same way. Plateaus are natural because as you decrease body fat, you may proportionally increase lean muscle mass. Muscle weighs more than fat. This means weight is redistributing and your shape is changing, even though a scale may be indifferent. Intuitive tools keep you in sync with your body so you recognize natural physical patterns. As you notice your body responding to different foods, ultimately you use intuition to nurture and maintain your weight.

"Food plays an important part in proper nutrition, but what you do to your foods and what your body does about them is the final answer."[3] Dr. Hazel Parcells

Weigh yourself once a month if you want to see your range. Do it at the same time of day, on the same day of each month. For example, weigh yourself on the first Saturday of each month before you eat or drink anything. Use the scale, but don't bond with it. Trust your body.

The rest of the month, follow your gut. Notice how you feel. Take care of yourself. Be your own scale. When balancing intake of food with knowledge of what feels right, you're "weighing in" intuitively.

The intuitive scale is flexible because it responds to holistic needs. Patience and grace guide you to recognize stress, while other intuitive tools maintain the balanced connection between sensual pleasures and your intelligence.

If you wonder about an eating choice because it is loaded with sugar or because the portion is over the top, then rule of thumb is: use foresight to connect with how you will feel the next day about eating it. Balancing food that gives you energy and tastes good, along with dignity and foresight, is eating intuitively. It makes sense and protects you from abusive eating choices.

Respecting yourself includes checking-in with your body, mind and emotions non-stop and responding from this holistic perspective to achieve your goals. Curiosity, with grace, keeps choices non-judgmental and flexible. Depending on intuitive tools keeps you in the flow and in sync with your life.

Rules are created by circumstances and circumstances are always changing. That's why keeping a fresh perspective based on an awareness of what's occurring right now makes sense.

Intuitive eating is your commitment to stay in the present by staying clearly in tune with your body, heart and mind. It takes effort. The intuitive connection with honesty and self-respect makes it clear that everything worth having has a price. There are no free rides.

The Clock, The Big Rush: Don't be a slave to time.

If you're not hungry at dinnertime, don't eat. If you don't eat, but are worried that you may be hungry later, then have a plan. Plan to eat a small healthy meal, perhaps a salad or fruit, or roast chicken with a green vegetable at least two hours before you go to sleep. This way, your food has time to digest before you go to bed and you won't wake up hungry in the middle of the night. If you do wake up hungry, visualize your healthy body as you drink a glass of water and go back to sleep.

If you had a big lunch, and are not hungry for dinner but have plans to go out, try this:

- While others enjoy their meal, order a light appetizer like a salad or a side order of a vegetable to eat as your main course. Based on curiosity and prudence, order what feels right for you. This is a personal decision. Connect with dignity when you order.

- Be social. Don't focus on food or on talking about your meal choice, unless someone asks, "Is that all you're having?" Then say "Yes" and smile, and change the topic. Stay in the present, which is about enjoying the company of others.

- Then EAT SLOWLY. By eating slowly you'll have more time for conversation. You can share what's on your mind, events of the day or some gossip.

- Put your fork down when you speak. This prevents unconscious eating.

- Take a deep breath between bites when you eat.

- Notice the fragrances, flavors and quality of your meal. Enjoy it.

- By you eating slowly, you and everyone at the table will be comfortable eating their meal. Importantly, you will be honoring your body, emotions and self.

- Don't finish early. Eating slowly gives your body time to be physically comforted by recognizing it's getting fed. If you don't make a big deal about what you are eating, no one else will. This reduces stress.

- Mindset becomes behavior because it's our attitude. When you eat with others, if you are uncomfortable with your choices, others at the table will be uncomfortable with you. Intuitive tools keep you comfortable by balancing your mindset.

Don't be bullied by the rush. A time crunch can create stress, making us feel the need to wolf down a meal - or starve! If you're in a time crunch and are hungry, resist your inner drama queen.

Eat half of the sandwich/portion/cup of soup now, enough to satisfy immediate hunger pangs, and save the rest until you have more time or are hungry later. You'll discover that eating slower is more satisfying than eating more quickly. You may learn that eating half will satisfy you enough to be comfortable until dinner.

Habits of eating on the run or eating very fast are a disconnect from the body and feel bad. Eating right does not take more time. It takes connecting with intuitive tools to recognize choices that feel dignified, emotionally and physically.

There is an expression: 'Penny wise, pound foolish'. When you eat sitting down, you eat less and when you eat slowly, you eat less. Don't buy into the bondage of time stress with your eating habits.

Intuitive eaters feel pressure of time crunch and depend on using the "pause" to maintain a clear perspective. Patience, foresight and curiosity enable us to avoid bondage to food choices that although convenient, make us feel bad afterwards.

Common Challenges

These common challenges can be overcome by eating intuitively:

- **Convenience eating-** It may appear eating on the run nurtures your body, but the digestive system is more efficient when you eat in a calm way, plus, you get more energy from your food.[4] When possible, organize the day so you sit down to eat. That way you'll notice food with all the senses, reconnect with your intuitive voice and actually be calmer for the rest of the day.

- **Habitual eating** - When under time constraint, habit may be to fall into an old pattern of emotional eating or mindless noshing. This is being in the matrix. Use the tools to break out.

- **Ignorant eating** - is a disconnect from your intuition. Because you are not connecting with your body, it may store the food as fat or rebel with poor digestion, which means less nourishment and no satisfaction. Use your senses to notice what you're eating and connect with your body.

To shelve self-defeating habits, connect with your 5 senses and depend on intuitive tools. Use curiosity to experiment with eating. Notice how your body feels and reacts to the pressure of time. Use patience and tenacity to be good to yourself.

Eating with tenacity has long term holistic rewards including:

- Peace of mind.

- Feelings of physical harmony, including a healthier body.

- Long-term benefits you feel that show all over.

- Satisfaction with yourself.

The Media Manipulates Minds

The average American sees 3,000 ads a day.[6] Commercial media has one goal, which is to get us to buy. What's being sold for our body is usually a stereotyped image that is not realistic and often not real. Body image flashed in front of us as ideal isn't, but the impact on us is real and it's enslaving.

The Media Awareness is a site for parents and teachers that focuses on media body stereotyping and media violence and its impact on us at

media-awareness.ca/english/issues/stereotyping/women_and_girls/women_beauty.cfm

The reasons for manipulation are economic. The website states:

"The stakes are huge. On the one hand, women who are insecure about their bodies are more likely to buy beauty products, new clothes, and diet aids. It is estimated that the diet industry alone is worth anywhere between 40 to 100 billion (U.S.) a year selling temporary weight loss (90 to 95% of dieters regain the lost weight).[5] On the other hand, research indicates that exposure to images of thin, young, air-brushed female bodies is linked to depression, loss of self-esteem and the development of unhealthy eating habits in women and girls."

About-Face is a site whose mission is "to equip women and girls with tools to understand and resist harmful media messages that affect self-esteem and body image." It has a "gallery of offenders" that shows popular ads and articles and points out how they are artificial, as well as having a helpful "resources" tab. Find out what's real. Don't be a slave to the images of media. **about-face.org/**

The Rules, Peer Pressure

Intuitive priority is to treat yourself with dignity and respect and it happens by being honest with yourself. You're not bound to anyone's point of view about what, when or how you should eat. You're bound to your body, heart, mind and soul. If friends are addicted to fast food, that's their choice. If this puts too much temptation in your way and you're wavering, then re-examine your core values. Use intuitive tools to be true to yourself. Enjoy being you.

Bond with friends, but don't be a slave to peer pressure. Use foresight for self-defense when you make eating choices. How can you be tempted by something that you will regret the next day? Who wants to live in servitude? Who wants to live in the Matrix?

There are always alternatives. Use curiosity and tenacity to find them. If you are with buddies who you know are going to make a quick stop at a drive-through, laugh. Hug yourself, and admire the fact that you have courage and trust your intuition. As long as you feel good about yourself, you're making the right choices. Be flexible and smart for you. What other people eat is their business. What you eat is your business.

For everyone, eating is personal. Depend on your internal support system 24/7. The natural choice is be healthy and eat what works for your body, stress and lifestyle. Depend on your tools to do the right thing and be your own boss.

Being intuitive is enjoying free will. Free will means you're not born to be a slave to anything. Intuitive free will leads to choices for the best overall quality of life. Intuition never leads to things that are destructive or deceitful to yourself or others. Depending on intuitive tools to stay connected to free will, maintains the comfort of balance and self-control.

This is your life. Eating well is a personal responsibility and pleasure. Don't be pacified by a scale, subdued by time or coerce yourself into eating patterns that feel uncomfortable. Bondage creates obstacles by putting you in the matrix.

Stay aware of your intuition and you will stay out of the matrix. There are always options. Your ability to say no to certain things gives you the freedom to say yes to others.

Factoids:

For less calories when you're out with the crowd:

- Order half the amount of pasta with one-fourth the total sauce. Enjoy the flavor as you eat slowly.
- Order egg white omelets.
- Request your burger buns be grilled dry.

- Order lean roast beef instead of tuna salad (tuna salad is full of mayonnaise).

- Order fajitas without the butter poured on at the end - you won't miss the taste.

- Ask to have your salad served with half the amount of dressing, or have the dressing on the side so you can see how much you're getting, and then use prudence about how much to use.

- Ask to have your main dish served on a small plate.

- Share dessert with the gang.

- Eat soup or dessert with a teaspoon.

- Don't be a slave to eating habits.

Am I Really Hungry?

Chapter 22 : **Hedonism and Sensuality**

"If we had a better understanding of the signals our bodies send to our brains, might we take more pleasure from them?"[1]
New York Academy of Sciences

The movie 9 ½ Weeks has a scene in front of a refrigerator where Mickey Rourke feeds Kim Basinger strawberries and honey, which says, in much more than words, that eating is sexy. Often in movies and in literature, sensual eating is a prelude to an erotic scene. 6th sense eating brings out the intuitive hedonist in each of us. The traditional definition of hedonism is the pursuit of sensual pleasures as the highest good. An intuitive hedonist indulges in sensual pleasures, but she is not an extremist.

The intuitive eater is privately exquisitely appreciative of his or her life. It's intuitive to enjoy eating. It's sexy to have a healthy appetite and it's sexy to enjoy eating. Why not connect with your inner intuitive hedonist?

An intuitive eater chooses foods that satisfy hunger and pleases his senses. H may see food as a gift that supports his life or may see a plate of lasagna and think of his grandmother. The point is: the intuitive hedonist looks at what he or she is eating, does the pause to gain perspective (patience) and makes a pleasurable emotional connection with her food.

Mixing the pleasures of the senses with the pleasures of the heart and mind, takes the eating experience to a new level. This kind of pleasure is the difference between flying first class or coach. Sure you get there either way, but the difference is in the quality of the trip and ultimate pleasure of your ride.

Sensuality is exciting because it's stimulating. Our senses arouse us by signaling pleasure or a problem. Eating to the point of just being full is a delicious experience. Overeating is painful. Excess doesn't ultimately give pleasure. Instead, overeating creates an imbalance that is not intuitive.

Enjoying sensual pleasures of eating in moderation is sexy because it satisfies, but does not saturate. It leaves you clear-headed and feeling good inside and out. Moderation with eating leaves energy to pursue other pleasures.

Hedonistic eating is a choice. To enjoy a good meal, begin with a pause. Look at your plate, inhale aroma, admire it, anticipate flavor with your tongue and mind (memory), all in the blink of the eye, which is how long it takes the brain to make the connection and recognize or categorize these sensations. Then, bingo - it's sensual and that's exciting.

It can be a pleasure to sit down and relax while eating. If you have the responsibility of buying and preparing food, it's great to have someone else cook. I am always grateful to eat when I'm hungry, and usually say a silent, simple prayer of appreciation from my childhood. Even when out for a business dinner, I pause to say *Thank You* before eating, which relaxes me just enough to glimpse what's on the plate before I pick up my fork.

Pausing avoids mindless eating by providing time to notice what you're doing. It's a good eating habit and no one notices. We all have our own way of appreciating who we are and what we have. Your intuitive pause is a private moment.

Intuitive hedonism is the choice to experience your senses fully and with dignity. Looking at what you eat, admiring it and anticipating the enjoyment, is sensual. Using smell with taste sets the digestive system into high gear so the anticipation of the pleasure of satisfaction is magnified.

Pausing to really taste, smell and savor your food gives your stomach time to fully digest. It will take longer to eat and you will probably eat less than usual. Hedonistic pleasure is holistic.

It's nice to feel satisfied, not stuffed. Choose to not over-indulge, binge or starve yourself. Overindulging, binging and starvation cause discomfort. Discomfort is the opposite of pleasure.

To eat like a hedonist, explore what gives you pleasure:

- Depend on your tools and senses to recognize what gives pleasure and what doesn't. The physical sensations of hunger and needing to be satisfied come in degrees of intensity. Be flexible. Notice what you notice.

- The 5 senses sharpen our awareness of everything. They are natural pleasure assets. These gifts of sensuality are wasted when taken for granted, and pure hedonistic delight when recognized.

- People frame pictures for two reasons: first, it increases the intrinsic value of the art and second, it brings out the quality of an image. Life is a work of art framed by our environment. Using your senses to be aware of your environment when you eat, enhances your quality of life by sharpening awareness of messages you receive from your physical self.

To an extent, you're aware of your body, but not much. Of course, we all realize when we have to go to the bathroom. This is an urge everyone not wearing diapers recognizes and responds to. But do you know when you are thirsty? Are you clear about when you have had enough to eat? Do you recognize when food is spoiled or overcooked? Take time to notice yourself and what you feel physically. Learn about yourself.

Sensual eating is savoring food you eat for the pleasures it gives. It is the delicious way to eat. The intuitive pause is your moment to anticipate tasting your food. Eat slowly, chew more, and see how cool you are to be tuned into your 6th sense. Intuitive hedonism is a private victory over habit.

Enjoy everything:

- Breathe.

- Look at your food.

- See your food.

- See your environment. Look at the other people at the table. Share the pleasures of enjoying flavors and fragrances together.

- Smell the aroma.

- Tease yourself with anticipation.

- Have a small taste. How does it taste? Is it seasoned the way you like? Is it cooked the way you like? Is it crunchy, smooth, salty, sweet, warm, refreshing?

- Notice when you swallow your food. Is your body happy to receive it?

- Notice what makes you feel good. Use curiosity to find foods that enhance your libido and your life.

Enjoy eating, explore the limits of your sensuality:

- Try a taste of something new. A taste is just a mouthful - a rounded teaspoon. First, smell it. When you just taste something, the idea is to let it touch your whole tongue where there are taste buds to sense flavors. Since this is a taste, take your time and reflect on the sensation and flavor before you swallow.

- Have a plate with only a rounded teaspoon of different "tastes" on it, to practice using your intuitive tools while learning about yourself and also to reinforce self-control. And, it's a tease. Sometimes a tease can be just enough to satisfy. Learn what foods satisfy you.

- Smell and taste with your eyes closed. This sounds sexy, and it is.

- Play with your food and connect with your inner child. Try this when eating alone, or with a close friend or family member. Have fun exploring with your tongue.

- Learn how eating choices can give energy to live life fully, by noticing how different foods affect your day.

- Follow your curiosity about food and eating and see where it takes you. Discover something new about yourself.

- Appreciate your food and enjoy eating.

To discover your inner hedonist:

- Using all 5 senses helps you relax to enjoy the experience. Talk about what you sense to the person you're eating with, and share sensations.

- In learning to be a hedonist, don't be 'put off' by lack of experience. Appreciation is intuitive. Enjoy eating while respecting yourself, and the rest is easy.

- As intuitive eating becomes a pleasant habit, it takes the pressure off of 'deciding' what to eat and puts the emphasis on choosing what feels right. Try new experiences in small doses.

- Ease into new things one step at a time, always staying connected with intuitive tools. They are your protective guides. Change is natural, but not necessarily easy. The only way to try new things is protectively.

It's a challenge to work through inertia caused by unconscious bondage to inner dialogue. When you feel doubts raised by inner dialogue, use the tools to let go of imposed limits and recognize it's time to start a new conversation. Remember: all progress is good progress.

- Start now to eat intuitively. Procrastination is stressful. Use curiosity and courage to discover what you're eating, how it smells, tastes and feels. Find new sensations. It will be fun. Use teaspoons to tease yourself with tiny bites. Being playful is intuitive and relaxing.

- Stay true to yourself by depending on your inner voice. When you feel stress, pull the trigger and reconnect with your tool chest so that you feel protected. Every day has ups and downs. Some eating environments please, while others create stress.

- Stay clear about what works for you.

Traps that inhibit sensuality are formed without realizing it by mental and emotional patterns. Once you recognize these, you can release them by using your tools and 5 senses to stay clearly in the present.

"Nobody can go back and start a new beginning,
but anyone can start today and make a new ending."[2]
Maria Robinson

When we watch a group of whales or pack of wolves, each animal radiates a totality within themselves. Animals do not judge themselves. Instead, self-acceptance is natural in all animals. They exhibit patience with themselves and their young. For example, if you watch an animal learn to hunt, there is a calm attitude between the young and the old, and individually within each. This is instinctive behavior. Connect with your inner animal and patience, and enjoy yourself.

Intuition is a connection with your authentic self. When you enjoy what you eat, you are enjoying your whole self. The pleasure touches way beyond eating. It is a feeling of being complete.

Eating with others is a way of sharing pleasure. There was a chewing gum commercial, "Double your pleasure, double your fun..." Eating with others is also a way of enhancing your libido. Our senses are a connection to the erotic. When the topics of hedonism and sensuality come up, many immediately think of sexual pleasure.

Admiring food with a partner, smelling the aroma together, and tasting food together is sharing intimate pleasure. According to Dr. Alan Hirsch, an expert on our sense of smell, food aromas cause sexual arousal.[3]

We know from experience that smell is an emotionally loaded sense. Of course, this is not a big surprise. Many people consider foods a natural aphrodisiac. In fact, the most important thing you can do to boost your libido is eat a healthy diet and maintain a healthy weight. Intuitive eating is good for your libido! Let your imagination wander.

My experience is what makes a great sex life, in a long-term relationship, is having a great sensual life together. Sensuality warms us up for sexual seduction. Eating is incredibly sensual. Have you ever looked someone directly in the eyes while putting food in your mouth? Suddenly, eating together becomes intimate. Eye contact and eating are hot together. They are a sensual high.

When you eat with your partner and enjoy the intuitive pause to smell and taste and savor, you relax. Relaxing melts stress and the sensual experience is enhanced. You start to anticipate other pleasures and become playful as you enjoy your senses. Anticipation creates desires that are exciting.

Romantically, people think of sensuality as the beginning of eroticism. Sensual pleasures that connect with your whole body are an arousing tease. It can lead anywhere. Anticipation is exciting because it's about possibilities. If you are looking for that erotic or romantic encounter, eat to savor the pleasure.

Eating can be a wonderful way to develop, reaffirm or renew romantic bonds. This is especially true if you eat until you're just full, so you will have room for a special dessert.

The Intuitive Hedonist's tool chest:

Prudence is weighing options to choose foods most pleasing and most nurturing.

Dignity gives you a sense of deep satisfaction.

Curiosity discovers pleasures of appearance, aroma and taste that are aroused and satisfied.

Patience relaxes you to enjoy eating, physically and emotionally, and reduces stress between your mind and body.

Courage is trying new eating experiences, being playful and trusting yourself and your enjoyment.

Tenacity and **Determination** are the intuitive way to protect and honor yourself.

Self-discipline means eating so your body is just satisfied, not stuffed.

Grace is an attitude of appreciation and kindness.

Foresight reminds you that food gives energy, maintains sexual hormones, sparks emotional bookmarks of love and is associated with sexual arousal. It also protects by helping you be aware of personal boundaries.

There are many photos online of figs, strawberries, asparagus, caviar, peaches, and bananas that are full of double entendres. Foods have suggestive shapes, arousing aromas, feel sensual in your mouth, and at the same, time provide energy. Explore the variety with someone you love. Some foods, like chili peppers, raise body temperature and champagne tickles your nose.

Food energy is sexy because all productive energy is exciting. The more energized you are, the more alive you feel. Be an intuitive hedonist. Get the most out of life.

Factoids:

Foods increase male and female sex hormones, elevate mood or boost sperm production. Importantly, foods play a vital role in increasing our blood flow. Many foods stimulate our nervous and circulatory systems, ultimately sending more blood flowing to our sex organs, resulting in enhanced sexual arousal and performance.[4]

- Watermelon has the amino acid citrulline in it, which relaxes blood vessels, which results in increased blood flow throughout our body.

- Dark chocolate contains serotonin, which boosts our mood, and phenylethylamine, which mimics the brain chemistry of a person in love.

- Celery contains natural plant estrogens.

- Oysters contain zinc, which is essential for producing testosterone, and boosts dopamine, which governs brain activity, and increases sexual desire for men and women.

- Wild Salmon and other cold-water fish (sardines, herring, trout, etc.) are high in omega-3 fats, which helps increase overall health and sexual stamina. Omega-3s are also critical to the brain and nervous system. Additionally, they improve mood, memory and brainpower.

- Other foods that boost your libido include: pumpkin seeds, eggs, shrimp, lean proteins like wild boar and poultry, garlic and peanuts.

Remember to use your sensuous nose.

"It's interesting to note that the sounds we make during the arousal stage of love making are similar to the sounds we make in response to an appealing odor. You may lift the lid of a simmering stew and exclaim, "ahh" or "ooh" and is the same sound you make when your lover strokes an erotically sensitive part of your body."[5]

Dr. Alan Hirsch, MD, FACP, Neurological Director of the Smell and Taste Treatment and Research Foundation in Chicago

Am I Really Hungry?

Chapter 23 : **Satisfaction**

"Arriving at one goal is the starting point to another."[1] John Dewey

Satisfaction is a feeling of achievement. It's a process, not a state of being. As you practice using intuitive tools, sound bites of satisfaction happen. You don't know how the adventure will turn out, but do know you'll learn about yourself and what you need to have for the best quality life, and that's satisfying. Use your imagination and plan to succeed. Satisfaction comes with effort and commitment.

The imagination is where you create what you wish to be real. By allowing yourself to imagine or dream, you create room in your life for these to happen. Imagine being automatically connected with your tools and in sync with yourself. You are a healthy, happy weight and like the way you eat. Of course, life demands more than our imagination; however, the imagination is a vitamin for self-discipline and hard work. Let yours work for you.

When we create something, we always create it first in a thought form. If we are basically positive in attitude, expecting and envisioning pleasure, satisfaction, and happiness, we will attract and create people, situations, and events which conform to our positive expectations."[2] Shakti Gawain

Life is an adventure that may not turn out the way we anticipate, but it's worth the challenge of being true to yourself. Consider the alternative. This adventure includes trying unfamiliar foods and eating habits. It's natural to feel a little frightened when you don't know what will happen. You may get off to a fast start, fall down and have to begin again. Patience maintains perspective, and tenacity keeps you focused on goals. Trying something new is bold. Holding fast to your truth brings satisfaction.

Facing a challenge requires courage, determination and tenacity. Nobody can understand how you feel because nobody is you. Still, amazingly, as you use intuitive tools to focus on healthy eating, support comes from others.

People are attracted to someone who has an attitude of moving ahead in life based on her values. It's inspiring. When you accept a challenge and give it your best no matter the odds, you get a sound bite of satisfaction.

Each of us has unique metabolic and hormonal make-up as well as unique stress. This means you aren't always satisfied by what may satisfy someone else. Your needs and tastes are different so a satisfying meal will also be different.

Physical and emotional satisfaction around eating grows, as patience lets you know and trust yourself during the trial and error of learning to listen to that little voice. Satisfaction from following through becomes a comfortable, gentle feeling of balance.

We are built to conquer environments, solve problems, achieve goals, and we find no real satisfaction or happiness in life without obstacles to conquer and goals to achieve."[3] Maxwell Maltz

When a meal is not satisfying, be curious. Pause for perspective and examine options to recognize what's causing frustration. Life isn't fair, but that doesn't mean you can't be fair with yourself. Use grace and you always have the choice to succeed. Ultimately, life gives balance when we allow it.

Sometimes you may be satisfied by a meal, but not with other things in your life, and confuse that with hunger. Be curious about what drives you and be honest with yourself. It's satisfying to protect yourself from destructive eating.

Confusion is an uncomfortable feeling of being out of balance with yourself. It's the 6th sense nudging you to remember or realize something. To clear up confusion, use the tools with your 5 senses to connect with what's happening in your environment and get back on track with yourself.

Two examples: (1)Tenacity and determination connect with a memory of the last time you ate something and it didn't satisfy, so you become aware that you eat certain foods only out of habit. (2)You take an intuitive pause, redirect your energy to decide if you're hungry or not, and recognize you feel pressure to eat. It's not satisfying to eat because of pressure or when your body isn't hungry. It's uncomfortable.

Inner dialogue pushes emotional buttons and throws a smokescreen over what's real, so we eat because we feel sorry for ourselves. For example, my friend B took herself out to dinner and noticed couples and families at other tables. Inner dialogue said she was a social failure. To compensate, B ate the entire basket of bread and ordered way too much food. Ouch!

Inner dialogue is a trap that sabotages satisfaction. It's a glass ½ empty attitude of defeat that creates fear and doubts. When you notice inner dialogue creating pangs in your enjoyment of a good meal, pull the trigger and find your inner voice.

Try this to find satisfaction when the going gets tough:

- Connect with dignity and courage.

- Use foresight as self-defense.

- Tap into patience to breathe and connect with your body, and pause.

- Use grace to see the glass as half full.

- Realize that you are amazing.

- The next time you're in a funk, treat yourself like a celebrity.

"Open your eyes, look within. Are you satisfied with the life you're living?"[4] Bob Marley

When doubt happens, turn to your tools. Pause for perspective at the first sign of going off-track. Use curiosity, dignity and grace to look at your mindset, and find satisfaction.

Perspective can give surprising insights that make us aware of habits that prevent satisfaction. For example, procrastination caused by personal laziness can be the core of unhealthy eating. Procrastination at mealtime is putting off responding to signals from your body. This disconnect is a habit leftover from being dependent on 20th century diets that teach not to take initiative when you're hungry!

Once you're aware of a self-defeating habit, it's easy to let it go. You'll discover soundbites of satisfaction from connecting with your whole self. Then, your self-control connects with self-respect and becomes automatic because satisfaction reinforces success.

"One of the great undiscovered joys of life comes from doing everything one attempts to the best of one's ability. There is a special sense of satisfaction, a pride in surveying such a work... The smallest task, well done, becomes a miracle of achievement."[5] Og Mandino

Sometimes a meal that you know is healthy is not satisfying, or you're hungry an hour later. I have had this happen and it is very frustrating. I have learned this means I'm in a nutritional rut.

Because the body's needs are always in flux, even 'healthy' eating habits can be eventually rejected. Being hungry after eating doesn't automatically mean you didn't have enough calories. Instead, it means the meal didn't satisfy your current physical need. The body, for its own reason, seeks something else.

Usually for me, this dissatisfaction happens abruptly because I tend to get into habits about what I eat. When this happens, at first it just drives me crazy and I start ransacking my apartment for stuff to nosh. Then, finally I pause and realize it's time for me to try different foods that nourish differently.

Intuitive eating is not about how much you eat that gives nourishment, but is about eating the types of food your body needs. Tune into your body. You will be glad.

Since your body is unique, experiment to find satisfaction. There are many kinds of proteins, vegetables and carbs. One protein may leave you hungry while another hits the spot. Use prudence and curiosity, with patience, tenacity, foresight and determination. When not satisfied after eating a "healthy" meal, it's time to choose other foods to eat.

"We need a variety of input and influence and voices. You cannot get all the answers to life and business from one person or from one source."[6] Jim Rohn

Even in a great romantic relationship, we learn that no one person can give us everything we need to be happy. It is the same with food. You cannot get all of the nourishment/satisfaction you need from eating the same food all the time. Eventually your body will just stockpile calories as fat, and you'll feel hungry. To feel satisfied, use curiosity and courage to try new foods. It's worth the effort.

Intuitive conclusions:

- Logically you want to have the most nutritious food because it's instinctive to give yourself and loved ones every opportunity to make the most of your lives.

- Any food that is really healthy and nutritious can be made tasty.

- Change is hard, but so what?! The alternative is having an unhealthy body and every disadvantage it brings. That's pretty bad.

- There is excellent food available at markets and food stores all over this country. There is wonderful variety served in restaurants. Eating intuitively helps you recognize what works for your body. Be curious.

Intuitive eating is easy. Use your 6th sense. The effort you put into it is reflected in the amount of satisfaction you get.

Use prudence to go wild with healthy alternatives. Have fun with variety, while learning about what feels good. For example, you may always eat chicken with a vegetable for dinner and believe this is the healthy, natural 'diet' for your body. Then, it happens that you're hungry an hour later. Your body is not satisfied.

The next meal, substitute lamb, beef or fish as your protein source. Eat a baked potato because baked potatoes are full of minerals. Baked sweet potatoes are even better. Variety is the spice of life that makes us feel complete (satisfied).

We tend to eat what we have always eaten, which is not helpful except to keep us alive. Choose to get the most out of being alive. Prudence, foresight and 5 senses, with the lessons learned in the school of life, make it clear that options are open. Choose to be aware.

A source of perpetual dissatisfaction for all of us comes from messages through mass media telling us how we should feel. Commercials focus our emotional buttons hoping to manipulate us to buy a product. Even though commercials and advertisements are elevated to an art form, we know they're often misleading. We're promised satisfaction and the product doesn't satisfy. Truth in advertising would be a great service.

Every day, you experience satisfaction that has nothing to do with eating. Still, every satisfaction connects with self-respect. Satisfaction comes in different ways. The list is endless, which is good.

List things that give you soundbites of satisfaction. Here is a start:

- Enjoying a meal and feeling satisfied afterwards.

- Learning about food that's good for your body gives the satisfaction of accomplishment.

- Receiving a compliment.

- Knowing you have done your best is the type of satisfaction that leads to peace of mind.

- You exercise and your body feels good.

- Doing what is right for your whole being brings satisfaction with yourself.

Please smile now. Feel satisfied with yourself for reading this - because you know you are changing your life.

"How often I have found that we grow to maturity not by doing what we like, but by doing what we should. How true it is that not every 'should' is a compulsion, and not every 'like' is a high morality and true freedom."[7] Karl Rahner

Tough Love (Parenting)

Intuitive eating is a lifestyle commitment. As parents, our choices impact our children. Usually, 'tough love' refers to parenting choices and responsibilities. Tough love is doing what is right, instead of what is easiest. As a mother, I know that it's easier to give a child what he wants to eat, than to say "no" and follow though. It takes energy (which burns calories) to do the right thing.

Ultimately tough love is satisfying, because it brings out the highest qualities in us and in those we love. Your 6th sense provides clarity and long-term perspective to make this choice, and intuitive tools connect with your inner strength to follow through. Tough love is true love.

Talking about using intuitive tools when you share meals with adolescent children, opens communication that rises above emotions. When kids realize that they are actually being heard, they're more careful about what they say. When parents stretch to communicate with their kids, they're able to let go of frustration and resentment that comes with the responsibilities of parenting.

Adolescents are interested in learning how to recognize signals that will give them advantages as they make life decisions and deal with peer pressure. Sharing mutual concerns may initially be a surprise, but teenagers are very aware that they're inheriting our world and hungry for ways to deal with it.

No matter how old or how young children are, they always look to us as an example of how to handle life's challenges. Speaking the truth is a powerful kind of love. Choosing to be honest with yourself and live life fully is great stuff. It's hard for children to learn to be self-reliant in our self-indulgent world. Being honest is a start.

Honest communication feels genuine and respectful, and builds trust. People instinctively respond to it. Your intuitive eating lifestyle is a commitment to being honest, real and staying in the present. Teaching this to your family will give you satisfaction for the rest of your life.

If your kids give you a hard time about the new eating lifestyle, laugh. Laughter is contagious. Keeping a sense of humor about eating relieves stress. With children especially, humor feels forgiving. Sometimes kids say or do things just for effect and when you laugh with compassion, it lets them laugh at themselves and gives you the opportunity to introduce your perspective about eating or nutrition without stress or guilt.

Importantly, laughing together is a way of enjoying each other and releasing tensions. When you talk about intuitive tools, be sure to mention laughing is healthy. New things are easier to accept when we can laugh together about them.

When you connect with your safe place to use intuitive tools, you take full responsibility for your choices and for the direction of your life. What a great example for your kids! This is satisfaction.

The impact of communicating with children about your choices and eating struggles lets them know that you respect them, and that you respect yourself. This guides them to respect themselves. Another bonus is that it opens the door for your children to share their choices and struggles with you. Communicating teaches your children not to give up.

You want your kids to have every opportunity to succeed in life. It's good to be clear that you don't want them to fall through cracks because of ignorance or a lack of energy. Your example teaches curiosity and prudence, and feeding them what makes sense gives energy and health.

- Create a "Try Everything Once" rule to encourage your children to be curiously bold, but to do it with prudence, in moderation. A taste is just a teaspoon. Ask them to be creative. You may find yourself tasting ketchup on a spoon or biting into a raw potato in the name of curiosity. Teaching them intuitive tools encourages your children's personal freedom with food, because this teaches that they are in control of their eating choices.

Children easily relate to the tools because they instinctively search to make sense of life. Younger children, especially, are always very curious because it is intuitive to want to know the truth. Teenagers are searching for answers to questions about the smartest way to deal with life and the world they're inheriting. Talking about intuitive tools and sharing eating goals with the kids, says you have confidence in their abilities to think. It also lets them feel they too, can control things. That makes kids feel a little safer in our scary world.

Sharing your determination to tell yourself the truth validates your children's truth. It also teaches them self-respect and self-reliance. Sharing the process of intuitive eating tells your children that they hold the key for their own successes in life. Introduce your family to intuitive eating and explain they each have a safe place in their being with their own intuitive tools.

"Laziness may appear attractive, but work gives satisfaction."[8]
Anne Frank

Family Guide

Guide your family to access intuitive connections by talking about your eating values and goals.

- Let them know that you're involved and concerned with their decision making process.

- Connect them with protective messages they get from their senses 24/7.

- Tell them to follow their inner voice, knowing that it will never be self-destructive. For example, if they think their intuition is telling them they need to eat an entire box of cookies or to smoke pot - they are lying to themselves. Be clear about the importance of being deeply honest with yourself. Mention self-sabotage caused by lying.

- Let them know that you are aware advertising can be confusing or misleading. Talk about it. You'll be impressed by what children observe.

- Experience proves that ultimate satisfaction has to come from within. We all hold the answers to our own questions. Use your intuitive tools.

- Let your children know you hold the highest expectations for them.

Set a family standard based on the intuitive tools.

Curiosity is a value that opens doors for thinking.

Prudence teaches being alert to opportunities.

Tenacity is being true to yourself. It is inner strength.

Dignity builds pride and nobility.

Determination is a weapon against laziness and ignorance.

Patience reminds you that it's helpful to step back and take a deep breath in and a deep breath out, especially when you feel confused or frustrated.

Foresight is intuitive self-defense, an important way to protect yourself.

Self-discipline is important for being honest with yourself and shows self-respect, which is part of being dignified and makes choices clear.

Courage is always available when you need it.

Grace is to treat yourself with kindness and respect.

Serve your family what's healthy. Always be flexible about meals because that's how to stay in the present with your children and yourself.

- Set short term goals.
- Recognize growth.
- Relax by using your tools with yourself and your kids around eating.
- Show your kids how to relax around eating by using their tools.

As you use intuitive tools to focus on doing what feels right, it's natural to find satisfaction in eating.

"Personal satisfaction is the most important ingredient of success."[9]
Dennis Waitley

Factoids:

- Cinnamon, which we often have on cookies and other sweets, is a delicious gentle addition to tomato sauce as well as curry recipes. I have added a little cinnamon to my scrambled eggs and discovered they taste like custard. Add a shake to your vegetable soup and see the smiles.

- Studies show cinnamon can improve insulin sensitivity and blood sugar control. According to Dr. Richard Anderson, who did a study at the USDA's Human Nutrition Research Center, cinnamon seems to make insulin more efficient at taking glucose out of your blood and converting it to fuel in your body.[10] It is also a mood elevator.

- Over the past 30 years, the plates, cups, glasses, and utensils have gotten much bigger. In the 1960's, a dinner plate was about 8 ½" in diameter. Today your plates are 12" in diameter. A 9" plate holds about 140 calories and a 12" plate holds about 350 calories.[11]

- We are visual by nature. Big plates encourage overeating because they make the portions look smaller. Use 9" plates to serve your meals. Then, your family can put on the plate exactly the portion that is smart and satisfying. If you encourage them to look at their food, they will learn to recognize healthy portion size.

Teach your children to recognize what they notice with their senses. It will protect them throughout their lives.

"Cheese for breakfast, gold. Cheese for lunch, silver. Cheese for dinner, lead." Tuscan saying

Am I Really Hungry?

Chapter 24 : **Fashion, Media and Diets**

"I don't design clothes, I design dreams."[1] Ralph Lauren

Fashion and the desire to look and be attractive is part of being human. Fashion and media have huge impact on the way we see our bodies. Media clearly leads us to believe that image is the same as self worth. Mass media is powerful and expert at manipulating emotions. In Aesop's fable "The Wolf in Sheep's Clothing", the moral is "Appearances are deceptive." When we disconnect from intuition, we forget this.

Even in the Garden of Eden, there was a sense of fashion. Adam would place a flower in Eve's hair and Eve would decorate Adam's chest with a blueberry dye while they ate berries in the woods. Decoration of the body was a celebration of the soul. In the Garden of Eden, fashion was sublime. But, like all fashion, it went out of style.

The original purpose of fashion is to show respect for the beauty of your whole package. Your whole package is body, mind and heart. Clothing yourself is a form of courtship with your body. It's a seductive and personal way to express love. Originally, fashion was a form of sensuality. Many designers still see it that way.

"Today, fashion is really about sensuality—how a woman feels on the inside. In the '80s women used suits with exaggerated shoulders and waists to make a strong impression. Women are now more comfortable with themselves and their bodies—they no longer feel the need to hide behind their clothes."[2] Donna Karan

The idea that clothing is a form of fetish has nothing to do with dieting, but can be linked to intuition and our senses. Modern fashion is about feeling attractive. Success is sexy and looking fashionable has become a symbol of success. Plumage, the feathers on birds, is a kind of natural fashion statement used to identify and attract. Ideally, we dress intuitively to identify who we are and to attract others.

The earliest dieters were trying to gain weight! When the Rev. Sylvester Graham created Graham crackers for their high fiber content in 1829, this was the beginning of dieting. Since beauty and health were signaled by a full figure, the fashion trend in those days was plumper bodies. Sensually voluptuous, Lillian Russell was one of our most famous actresses at the turn of the 20th century and women wore padded clothing to look like her.

In the early 1900's, the fashion trend to identify with and attract the admiration of others was the hourglass silhouette. It was a mature woman's silhouette. Women wore a rigid boned corset called the "S BEND" corset. It was laced so tightly, women's hips were thrust back and their soft bosom forward forming the shape of a high-breasted bird called the pouter pigeon.

My grandmother was born in 1896 and got married 1916. Unfortunately, my grandmother had a naturally slender physique, which would have rocked in the 21st century, but was woefully out of step with the fashion of her times. As a result, my grandmother wore hip padding, stomach padding and bosom padding when she got married. According to family lore, on their wedding night, my grandfather was "very disappointed."

Lulu Hunt Peters, a Los Angeles physician, introduced the concept of calories with her book, Diet and Health with a Key to the Calories, published in1918. Based on her experience losing weight, it became a bestselling nonfiction book in 1923. Lulu Peters connected with her core intuitive tools. Besides calorie counting, her book's clear message is dieting can be a tough road to follow at times, and that self-discipline and willpower are key to winning the war against fat.

In the roaring 20's, the shape to identify with was sleeker. Limbs were exposed for the first time and dresses were shorter - usually mid calf. Women with large breasts bandaged their breasts to flatten them. The Symington Side Lacer was a bra designed to flatten the chest.[3] Ouch.

"A fashion is merely a form of ugliness so unbearable that we are compelled to alter it every six months."[4] Oscar Wilde

In the 30's, fashions became softer. Rounded breasts and waistlines gently reappeared. The natural variety of body types was appreciated. Physical fitness was considered important and sports wear for women was produced for the first time. At this time, *The*

Hollywood Diet, a short-term fad diet, was introduced. It would later become known as the Grapefruit diet, popular in the 1970's.

In fashion magazines, woman were urged to look at their shape, and then suggestions were offered as to which way to wear the style of the day that would be most flattering. Evening clothes were draped to hang in a curving or twisting way that gave women freedom of movement, as well as an elegant look.

"The dress must follow the body of a woman,
not the body following the shape of the dress."[5]
Guy de Givenchy

The 40's brought WW2 and with it, rationing of fabric as well as food. "Ideal Weight" charts were introduced. These matched weight with gender, height and frame. The style was padded or puffy shoulders, which mimicked a military look. Broad shoulders accented waistlines and they became more fashionable. With the boxy look, women wore dresses at a shorter length - right below the knee. WW2 ended in 1945. By the end of the 40's, the trend was for fuller, fitted shapes and longer skirts, often to mid calf.

Until the 1950's, teenagers generally dressed to look like their parents. Then, in the 1950's, fashions took a dramatic turn as our consumer driven society went into full action. By the end of the 50's, the fashionable shape was no longer the mature woman. For the first time, media, as a creator of fashion, was more important than anything else.

Diet pills based on amphetamine derivatives became popular. Since the second half of the 20th century, television, magazines and music continue to have a major impact on fashionable self-image.

Weight Watchers was born in the 1960's at the apartment of Jean Nidetch. She had been trying to lose 20 pounds for years, but always gained it back. She created a group environment with friends for support and diet advice. Ms. Nidetch was tenacious and used prudence to create an environment to maintain healthy weight through healthy eating habits.

Jean Nidetch connected to her intuitive tools. She used curiosity for a flexible approach to solve a problem she had been experiencing for years. She used patience and kindness with herself, to pause and discover her solution. She used grace to forgive her disappointment about not losing those 20 stubborn pounds. And she stayed connected with dignity. Determined, self discipline - with foresight and courage, she created an industry and kept her weight off.

Diet became a fad word in 1963 with the introduction of 'Diet Coke'. During the second half of the 20th century, with the blossoming of the diet industry, the body became viewed as a commodity. In the 60's, personal fashion became a political statement. It was a wave of fashion freedom represented by innovation in lifestyle and morals, as well as how to dress. Baby boomers, who were mostly college age, became the major consumer force.

In 1966, Leslie Hornby, known as Twiggy because she was stick thin, took the fashion world by storm. Her image became what the fashion world was all about. She was 17 years old, well managed and made nearly as much money as The Beatles, who also hit the world by storm in the mid-60's. Twiggy was on the covers of ELLE, Vogue, Harper's Bazaar, Look, Life and Newsweek magazines.

After four years, Twiggy dropped out of the very glamorous world of modeling to pursue a more 'ordinary' life. When asked why, she said, "You can't be a clothes hanger for your entire life!" She used foresight and dignity with courage, to connect with intrinsic self-respect, and was able to stay connected with her intuitive clarity. Also, since she was the first teenage icon, Twiggy was lucky that her "handlers" didn't look at her as a cash machine, and this enabled Twiggy to maintain her intuitive connection with herself.

In the 70's as social pressure to be stick thin became common, the eating disorders anorexia and bulimia became public. The phrase, made famous by Wallace Simpson, "You cannot be too thin or too rich" became a mantra, and diets skyrocketed in popularity. Diets of the 70's included The Atkins Diet and The Pritikin Diet. The diet drug "Fen-Phen", which ultimately was linked to heart valve damage, was popular. People were so busy listening to media about dieting, they didn't listen to their own bodies.

In the 80's, Princess Diana emerged as the fashion icon for the 20th century. It was well publicized that she dieted to lose weight and worked conscientiously to maintain her svelte appearance. It was also widely rumored that Princess Diana was bulimic. Was she a fashion victim? Are you?

"The goal I seek is to have people refine their style through my clothing without having them become victims of fashion."[6]
Giorgio Armani

Oprah Winfrey, one of our most respected public figures, is also a public dieter. In the 80's, she lost almost 70 pounds on a popular liquid diet and since then, her battles with eating have been well-documented. Oprah is a world mover and a shaker at hyper speed. She's a heroine of our culture. It's not easy. But, it is cool and we all want to be like her. We all want to feel the respect.

For Oprah to be her healthy weight, she has to find, make or take time for herself to do the pause. She has to renew her commitment to keep that connection. When we look at her life, it appears Oprah stays connected to her intuitive voice 95% of the time. We know this because of her dignity and courage.

Oprah quotes a letter sent to her by Marianne Williamson regarding losing weight, *". In fact, if you diet and lose weight, your mind will either put the weight back on or trip up in some other area. In order to lose weight on a permanent basis, you want a shift in your belief about who and what you are."*[7].

I believe when Oprah connects to her safe place and uses her core intuitive tools to connect 100% with her whole, holistic being, her amazing, impressive, personal strength will guide and support her to maintain her healthy weight, naturally.

Fashion trends, media and technology all impact self-image. Because life is so complex, because our 5 senses are simultaneously categorizing awareness at the rate of time, because we are thinking faster and doing more, everyone - no matter if we are man, woman or child – every one of us is part of a new kind of mind expansion. We're exercising a stealth muscle. That stealth muscle is the brain. And, it is burning calories. Of course, everything we do burns calories.

There was a study done in Russia where they had two groups of people take a relaxed walk through a park. For one group, they placed sculptures along the way; for the other, it was a typical park walk. The group that noticed the sculptures burned more calories.[8] They really used their eyes.

By intentionally focusing on what we see, hear, smell, taste and touch, we expand energy and burn calories. This means when you want to burn calories, but are too tired to move, you can do it with your senses. Be sensual and burn calories! Use self-respect and patience and have fun.

In the past, life moved at a slower pace. Generally. people learned skills and knew what to expect by the time, by the time they were 21 years-old. Thinking was more fixed. Now, we are learning at the speed of computer technology. That is burning calories. The ideas in this book are burning calories because they are things you have never thought before, and now you are digesting them.

This learning to be an intuitive eater is a total body/mind experience that becomes natural. You are learning and using new tools - you are not just learning ideas. Always learning burns calories.

Fashion is an idea. Ideas are a different kind of food, but one that you still use intuitive tools to properly digest. Fortunately, the fashionable style in the 21st century is the look of good health. This is right in tune with intuitive goals. One might say connecting with intuitive eating to stay healthy, strong and live the best quality of life, is fashionable.

Long ago, we dressed to decorate and honor our body. Now, we are in the habit of using our body to be fashionable. It is an intuitive disconnect when we measure self-worth by an image. Recognizing you're more than a body image, and staying in tune with your values, is self-respect.

"I am not looking like Armani today and somebody else tomorrow. I look like Ralph Lauren. And my goal is to constantly move in fashion and move in style without giving up what I am."[9]
Ralph Lauren

Hero worship of celebrity images inspires people to obsess about weight loss. Instead of relating to our body, values and life, we relate to celebrities and without thinking, want to look like them. It's a disconnect from our intuitive self.

"Fashion is what you adopt when you don't know who you are."[10]

Quentin Crisp

Sensuality is a kind of fulfillment. It is "being pleasing or fulfilling to the senses."[12] This a time, when we are so alive, that we connect with life and to each other with all our senses. It's happening because we intuit information faster than we can think. We're naturally sensual.

Our senses and mind are the ultimate gifts housed inside of our bodies. That's one reason why fashion is so important to us.

"Begin to see yourself as a soul with a body rather than a body with a soul."[11] Wayne Dyer

In our world, we are hit left and right about how to eat and what to wear. Eating is exciting. Being healthy is sensual. Sometimes when people dress attractively, we say they have good "taste". Dress in fashions that feel good to you and reflect your "taste", and enjoy eating. Trusting your intuitive voice is very sexy. When you feel sexy, you are sexy.

Factoids:

Media, driven by economics, has made us eat more by saying that bigger is better. 20 years ago, bagels were 3" in diameter; now they are 6" and the size of a slice of pizza has more than doubled. Big packaging encourages us to eat more.

Brian Wansink, PhD, author of Mindless Eating, conducted an experiment where his team randomly gave moviegoers either a medium or large size popcorn for free. The only rule was, no sharing.

After the movie, the team collected the containers to see how much people ate. It turned out that people with the large container ate 53% more than those who ate out of smaller container! Use foresight and buy smaller containers of food. Otherwise, you may end up wearing that gallon jug of mayonnaise.

If you want to lose 10 pounds, go to the store and look at a 10 pound bag of potatoes. Really look at it. Lift it, and feel what it's like to carry around. Now, imagine it leaving your body. Feel lighter.

If your goal is 20 pounds, do the same thing with a 20 pound bag of potatoes. Tenacity and self-discipline work with your senses to see and feel how to maintain your healthy weight.

Chapter 25 : **The Lucky Ones**

Today, all over our world, children and adults will die from starvation. Extreme hunger is a reality of our time. It has been said that as long as there is hunger in the world, there cannot be peace. I believe this.

"The war against hunger is truly mankind's war of liberation."[1]

John F. Kennedy

We are the Lucky Ones. While on our planet people must obsess about eating to stay alive, we have food from nearly every culture at our fingertips. It is glorious, from pizza to fried rice, hotdogs to sausage, spaghetti to curried shrimp, an English muffin to a baguette, we have choices. Our variety is priceless. No matter what the season, there is always ice cream and no matter what the reason, we can eat turkey or we can eat cake.

As you look at your body, you know it is composed of individual organs, rivers of blood, mountains of muscle, bacteria, bones, millions of cells, flesh, a brain, etc. You know when one organ is sick, like your stomach, the rest of your body doesn't function well. If you stub a toe, it can totally throw you off balance. Altogether, your body is a whole world. Importantly, your instinct when your body is ill or hurt is to heal it.

Our planet is a whole world. We are each part of the whole body of our world. Our gut tells us that our lives are connected with others so that we will recognize being part of a bigger picture. Instinct is to heal what's hurt. When people are hungry, we cannot have peace in our world. A hungry person cannot reason, because she is driven to do anything to survive. Because of hunger, our world is not healthy.

"A hungry man can't see right or wrong. He just sees food."[2]
Pearl S. Buck

In places where there is no choice about what to eat, people instinctively eat what their body needs. For example, poor people in southern United States have been known to eat the local clay soil. Why? Because it is unusually mineral rich and will nourish them! When circumstances are desperate, people intuitively eat what their body needs. You don't have to be desperate to eat what your body needs. But when you eat, you have to be honestly hungry and respect and recognize a physical need for nourishment.

In parts of Greece and Italy where there is poverty, people only eat - the highly regarded in our country - Mediterranean" diet. Why? Because olive oil, beans, unrefined cereals, fruits, vegetables and fish are readily available and so are moderate amounts of cheese, yogurt, meat and meat products. Also, anti-oxidant rich red wine is readily available and moderately consumed. There really is no other choice for these people. Because we have so many choices, we are the lucky ones.

With every blessing comes responsibility. Our blessing of food abundance gives us the responsibility of being tuned in and choosing wisely what we should eat. It also gives us a responsibility to help feed those who are hungry.

Constantly thinking about dieting or criticizing your physical image, is an unbalanced negative focus on weight that creates feelings of isolation. This self-critical habit becomes a vicious non-productive cycle and you feel lousy. One way to turn obsessing about food and eating into a positive and productive part of your life, is to think about food needs of others.

"Most of our citizenry believes that hunger only affects people who are lazy or people who are just looking for a handout, people who don't want to work, but, sadly, that is not true. Over one-third of our hungry people are innocent children who are members of households that simply cannot provide enough food or proper nutrition. And to think of the elderly suffering from malnutrition is just too hard for most of us. Unlike Third World nations, in our country the problem is not having too little – it is about not caring enough!"[3] Erin Brockovich

Tuning in to feeding the hungry throughout the world is as simple as pushing a button on your computer, or as involved as you want to be. You have the tools. With dignity and courage, see beyond yourself. Ultimately, you can feed social and emotional hunger by helping others. There is always balance. Broadening your perspective is the healthy way to embrace life. Being aware of everyday hunger in the world beyond your own three meals, lets you recognize and celebrate who you are.

"Personal transformation can and does have global effects. As we go, so goes the world, for the world is us. The revolution that will save the world is ultimately a personal one."[4]
Marianne Williamson

Eating intuitively for health and energy includes appreciating that food is nourishment for sustaining life. It's time to be more self-reliant in our self-indulgent world. With empathy, you can feel the hunger of others because you know your own hunger. Feeding those who are hungry, you are giving the gift of life.

Importantly, by feeding others, we create a ripple effect to help heal our world. It's about starting and letting momentum take over. Here are ways to begin:

feedingamerica.org

Feeding America used to be called Second Harvest. They have a food bank locator and up-to-date Hunger news. This excellent site offers all kinds of opportunities to get involved and interact with others.

bread.org

Bread for the world helps feed hungry people worldwide. It's easy to get involved. This is a wonderful international site where you can take action to help feed others. It also keeps abreast of the politics of hunger so that you can help to fight hunger by staying aware of assistance reforms or bills, and adding your voice.

mazon.org

Mazon means food in Hebrew. This Jewish-based organization collects food for local charities of all races, ages and religions and is committed to finding a long-term solution to end hunger internationally. Jeremy Piven and Michael Ian Black are donors and celebrity ambassadors. The site is very helpful, listing ways to be involved to nourish others.

feedthechildren.org

Feed The Children is an amazing and touching site that focuses on feeding children around the world, with an emphasis on rescuing abandoned children and a special focus on American children. They also provide food for families in need of nourishment. The site lists all kinds of opportunities to participate. Do it.

endhunger.com

"The End Hunger Network works with the entertainment community to create and support media projects, programs and events to raise awareness and generate action to end childhood hunger."

This program makes certain people are eligible can get food stamps from the government and is connected to various projects working to eliminate the plight of hungry children. The site has a button to push that lists ways to get involved or volunteer at local hunger organizations. You just supply your zip code. John Travolta, Jeff Bridges and Tim McGraw are advocates for End Hunger.

"35 million people in the U.S. are hungry, or don't know where their next meal is coming from. 13 million of them are children. If we discovered that another country was doing this to our children, we'd be at war."[5] Jeff Bridges

thehungersite.com

It doesn't cost anything, and a few minutes at The Hunger Site is a form of doing an intuitive pause. This site has been actively feeding people for FREE for over 10 years. Just a click provides a hungry person with food. It costs nothing to participate and does the world a lot of good. There is a tab on the hunger site that says Take Action! When you click on, you will see a list of ways to help others. Please check this site out and participate.

"About 24,000 people die every day from hunger or hunger-related causes. This is down from 35,000 ten years ago, and 41,000 twenty years ago. Three-fourths of the deaths are children under the age of five.

Famine and wars cause about 10% of hunger deaths, although these tend to be the ones you hear about most often. The majority of hunger deaths are caused by chronic malnutrition. Families facing extreme poverty are simply unable to get enough food to eat. ... It is estimated that one billion people in the world suffer from hunger and malnutrition."

Mercy Corp is a partner with The Hunger site. Mercy Corp works in the toughest places in the world where there are natural disasters, poverty and conflict.

mercycorps.org

"Mercy Corps' partnership with The Hunger Site translates into lifesaving assistance for people in tremendous need around the world. When you visit, click, and shop at this unique site, you're making the future a little brighter for families who need food in the world's poorest places." Dan O'Neill

Besides helping to feed others, the hunger site is a source of opportunities to:

- Provide mammograms - **nationalbreastcancer.org**

- Donate to causes related to children's health that are designed to connect people in simple ways to make the world a better place. **one.org** fights AIDS and extreme poverty; **hki.org** fights and treats preventable blindness; **pofsea.org** is a prosthetics outreach foundation

- Spread literacy - **roomtoread.org** works to break the cycle of poverty by teaching children to read; **firstbook.org** works to improve the quality of education for children nationwide.

- Save the rainforest - **worldlandtrust-us.org** buys land to preserve the rainforests

  nature.org/ The Nature Conservancy *"The Nature Conservancy's mission is to preserve the plants, animals and natural communities that represent the diversity of life on Earth by protecting the lands and waters they need to survive."*

  rainforestconservation.org *"The organization is working to expand the Reserva Comunal Tamshiyacu-Tahuayo in the Peruvian Amazon. This is to supporting 14 species of primates, the most ever recorded in this region.*

- Rescue animals - **fundforanimals.org** *The Fund for Animals operates four world famous animal care facilities, including the Cleveland Amory Black Beauty Ranch sanctuary in Murchison, Texas for abused and rescued animals, The Fund for Animals Wildlife Center in Southern California, the Cape*

Wildlife Center in Cape Cod, Massachusetts for the medical rehabilitation and treatment of injured wildlife, and the Rabbit Sanctuary for abandoned "pet" rabbits

petfinder.com/foundation provides relief in times of stress or disaster.

nsalamerica.org *North Shore Animal League America is a non-profit humane organization supported 100% by voluntary donations dedicated to finding the best possible home for each pet in its care, even if the pet is blind, deaf, or otherwise disabled. To date, the League has placed close to 1 million puppies, kittens, cats and dogs into carefully screened homes.*

projecthealthychildren.org

hki.org

vitaminangels.org

Micro nutrients that we have - like iodine in our salt, folic acid in our flour or zinc, iron and vitamin A, can be added to water or food supplies in other parts of the world to prevent devastating, lasting and expensive birth defects. Every minute, a child dies of malnutrition, and babies are born deformed, blind or painfully damaged because their mothers were malnourished when they got pregnant. These organizations work to change that by providing essential nutrients for healthy children all over the world. The three URL's above are organizations you can work with to change the fate of innocent children. You can be a life saver.

"A year's supply costs less than the cheapest hamburger...It's much cheaper to prevent birth defects than to treat them"[7]

There are many ways to help others:

shoe4africa.org

Using racing as a vehicle, shoe4africa provides food, medicine access to education and more. The support provided by this organization enables the people of Kenya to keep their Dignity. By doing this, they are empowering these people to rebuild their lives. This is beautiful. The site lists ways to participate.

Please watch these 2 clips. The first is about the Kenya's first public children's hospital, which shoes4africa is building, and the second is about dignity in a refugee camp. On both clips, dignity and courage radiate from the children.

youtube.com/watch?v=DeiuZ1fbdRM

youtube.com/watch?v=0qnHV5_IHXU

firstgiving.com and **justgiving.com** (UK)

"We exist to help you raise more money than you ever thought possible for the causes you care about. When we created the company in 1999, our dream was to enable any charity, however small, to use the web to raise money at very low cost."

onevillageatatime.org

The easiest way to help is to go to this website and make a donation. If schools want to participate, they can hold a fundraiser, such as a bake sale, to feed the children in Nambale. The school can then send the proceeds as a check to:

One Village at a Time
121 W. Newton St.
Boston, Ma.
Att: Susan B. Gross, Executive Director

mycharitywater.org

Right now, there are almost a billion people on the planet without clean and safe drinking water. Using mycharitywater.org, can help change that.

You can start a campaign to use your birthday; or create a competition to run, swim, walk or do just about anything to raise awareness and money for those in need. mycharitywater.org has a unique a fundraising model: 100% of all money raised goes straight to water projects. Every project is then proved with GPS coordinates and photos, and posted on Google Earth for you to see."

threesquare.org/

The vision of Three Square is simple: No one in our community should be hungry. By bringing together the resources, experience and passion of the people and businesses of Southern Nevada, we can make sure no one has to. When we work together, we don't just serve food. We serve hope.

The food bank serves as a central collection and distribution center for donated, rescued and solicited food and grocery product. We provide bakery, produce, dairy, non-perishable products and ready-to-eat meals to non-profit and faith based organizations who serve those in need in our community. We also facilitate childhood and senior nutrition programs.

Celebrity Chef Kerry Simon, whose mac and cheese comfort food recipe is in Chapter 27, holds threesquare.org very close to his heart. Despite his busy schedule, Chef Simon regularly fills backpacks on Friday afternoons so that local children, who would otherwise go hungry, can have food over the weekend. Go to the website to see how you can participate with or support Three Square.

mothersonamissionintl.com

Mothers On A Mission International is a group working together to mobilize others in helping underprivileged women and children.

We are restoring women and children to their dignity and destiny.
We are raising up young leaders in communities around the globe.
We are rescuing, restoring and rehabilitating street boys in Africa.
We are providing business opportunities and resources for community development.

Chef Dorian Bergen, whose recipe is in Chapter 27, is using her prestige and energy to support this group's work rescue street children, and to feed children and build an orphanage in Kenya. You can be a part of this, too. Click on the site and learn how.

Amazingly, you will discover there is always enough time to draw into your life exactly what feels right. Since life doesn't come with a manual, we don't know what we need. Being curious about the needs of others can shed light on your needs and your path. Opportunities and options appear. If you work in soup kitchens for one meal a week, you're channeling your personal concerns about eating to feeding others - and feel good about yourself.

This also gives insights into your emotional relationship with food. When you help others, it enhances your life in a way that creates wisdom. Wisdom becomes common sense.

In our world, we don't have a lot of spare time, but when you value curiosity and dignity, there is always enough time to do the right thing. I live in NYC, and sometimes when I'm rushing, I see a blind person bravely navigating the stairs into the subway or an elderly person unsuccessfully trying to hail a taxi. It takes less then a minute to help these people and it helps me stay connected with my 6th sense because it always – very quickly- feels right.

When we help the less fortunate, we recognize how lucky we are. When someone appreciates us, we pause to appreciate ourselves, usually without realizing it.

Perspective creates balance. Balance is that comforting feeling of being in control. By helping others, we are less self-centered and more balanced. And as you connect with others, you are enriched.

I read about a woman who keeps a grocery bag handy, and every time she loses a pound, she puts a pound of canned food into the bag. When she collects 10 pounds, she donates it to the community food bank. This is a creative to help others by using tenacity, dignity, patience and grace.

Our gut feeling is to be the best we can be, to live the best possible life. Eating intuitively gives energy and inspiration to help ourselves by helping others who are hungry. We are The Lucky Ones.

"The day hunger disappears, the world will see the greatest spiritual explosion humanity has every seen."[6] *Federico Garcia Lorca*

Am I Really Hungry?

Chapter 26 : Beauty and Balance

Beauty is multi-dimensional and not just skin deep. It comes through you. As you connect with who you are inside and strive to live to your fullest potential, you achieve lasting beauty by living your truth. Truth is a link to inner harmony. Beauty, like satisfaction, is a process, not a destination. Even the most beautiful people in the world work at being beautiful.

"Every time you see a beautiful woman, just remember, somebody got tired of her"[1]

When supermodel Christy Turlington was asked how she manages to keep a sense of balance in the whirl of celebrity,[2] she replied that discipline and personal dignity help her focus in her erratic lifestyle because they give her balance. Balance is a stress buster that lets natural beauty shine.

Every one of us lives with a swirl of relationships, responsibilities and physical realities. We all have erratic lifestyles. When you include the goal of being beautiful with your eating lifestyle and depend on the intuitive tools, inner balance and harmony make it clear that you have 'it'.

"When you are balanced and when you listen and attend to the needs of your body, mind, and spirit, your natural beauty comes out."[3] Christy Turlington

Turlington, a fashion icon, was asked what she learned from the world of fashion about a woman's relationship with beauty. She replied: *"Nothing. I think each woman has her own relationship to beauty... life teaches you.. about these matters, not modeling"*

Life teaches us about living. Enduring beauty is not found with the eye, but discovered by the heart. When you connect with all 6 senses, the holistic connection includes your unique inner beauty. It is beauty learned and recognized from the lessons of life.

Intuition is a kind of emotional intelligence that brings clarity by keeping us grounded. Being grounded keeps your perspective clear. For example, you see and smell a beautiful slice of chocolate cake and pull the trigger to connect with your 6th sense. Checking in physically you realize you're not hungry. Emotionally you love that beautiful cake and it even smells beautiful, but since you don't physically want or need it, you don't even taste it. This is self-discipline and foresight.

The beauty of this experience is visual and emotional. You feel great physically because you respected your body, and great emotionally because you're being good to yourself. This is dignity. You're in sync with yourself and this is beautiful.

Balance is a stress buster. It is a healthy perspective that opens doors to opportunities we need. Being balanced around eating brings feelings of control and physical comfort. This creates self-confidence, which is beautiful.

To achieve balance in eating includes breaking habits, leaving behind routines and learning what feels right. It includes noticing what isn't working now, as well as what never did work. Nothing worth having comes easily. Christy Turlington works very hard to maintain a positive mindset. She helps others through charity work. Importantly, Turlington respects herself as a person who is always evolving. Her lifestyle code is flexibility and balance.

> *"It isn't sufficient just to want - you've got to ask yourself what you are going to do to get the things you want."*[4]
> *Franklin D. Roosevelt*

Think of your life like the creation of a fabulous diamond. A diamond is formed over eons of time from patterns of stress and pressure - hot and cold, that begins deep inside the earth. Then it is mined. Next it's cut, polished and mounted. To be mounted, the diamond must be balanced, and then, finally it is recognized.

You are a diamond formed by the patterns of your history, the stress of your life, mined by lessons, and then cut by experience, polished by friends and foes and now you are ready to be recognized. It's time to find your balance.

In the search for beauty, our senses lead to balance by giving pleasure and protection. It's natural to recognize both sides for a clear perspective. This keeps us in tune with changes and in the present, by reminding that the only thing steady is the moment.

State of mind, flexibility and grace, in tune with your 5 senses, work in harmony to keep life balanced. But, trying times happen because we are always evolving. It's natural to feel frustrated and experience painful changes in the quest to know yourself.

"Pain is the breaking of the shell that confines understanding. It is the medicine of the physician of the soul that heals itself"[5]
Kahlil Gibran

Pain brings understanding and heals sickness. Things are not supposed to always be wonderful. As you make choices at mealtime, think of good health and this will bring you pleasures beyond the meal.

Use your inner hedonist to maintain perspective. See the big picture and live fully. Personal happiness is often a reflection of our physicality - health and beauty.

"The best part of beauty is that which no picture can express."[6]
Sir Frances Bacon, Sr.

Harmony is the opposite of stress. Being grounded creates feelings of harmony. Eating foods that enhance your body and spirit naturally create inner calm. Balance is harmony experienced by depending on your intuition. When you choose to be flexible and respect yourself, you're not fighting with your body and are at peace with yourself. This is beautiful.

Intuitive eating feels right because it's a spontaneous response to the environment and stress level. Rudy Reyes, a powerfully built charismatic ex-Marine, dedicated martial artist and actor was in NYC promoting his new book this week. We finished pre-taping a Joey Reynold's Show around midnight where I had been talking about intuitive eating, and Rudy noticed a table with corned beef sandwiches, pickles, etc. for the all-night show.

He connected with his body, stopped what he was doing to eat a sandwich and enjoyed it. Then, speaking of intuitive eating, he said, "You see, I saw that meat, bread and pickle and knew that was what my body needed." This is beautiful, and his body is too.

What makes us beautiful is when we know what we feel and need, and act on it! The tools of determination, dignity, foresight and courage are guides to depend on. It takes courage to refuse your own lies and courage to trust your truth.

It is when you're true to yourself that you shine. People sense it; some call it a light or charisma. Those who live their truth are beautiful.

Beauty is a holistic combination of qualities that put us at ease. We recognize it with mind, heart and senses. Enduring beauty is the energy of inner balance that radiates. It is exciting because beauty nourishes appreciation of life. Because it's grounding, you can connect with your natural beauty intuitively.

- Aromas and smells tantalize and invite, with promises that go beyond food. They create anticipation and beautiful memories.

- Follow your dreams. Notice dreams that electrify your senses. Excitement is a kind of passion that's beautiful.

- Create atmosphere. Music can lift, relax or recharge the spirit, and silence provides a refreshing rest. Quiet engages the senses to be more alert and offers a source of calm to see the beauty of your meal, your family, yourself.

- When stressed, our mouth gets tight and the area around our eyes gets tense. Taking time to reflect or pause leads to a sense of relaxation. As we relax, our features are able to resume their natural elasticity. So, take that pause before your first bite, and let your inner beauty show as you enjoy eating.

Balance and inner harmony are the result of respecting all aspects of who you are. Paying attention to what you sense, and depending on the tools, keeps you beautiful.

- Curiosity objectively and clearly emphasizes assets.

- Prudence shows options to consider to your advantage.

- Tenacity is being true to yourself, which creates inner harmony.

- Dignity keeps you neat, stylish, clean and feeling good.

- Determination is part of every choice you make.

- Patience is part of flexibility that relaxes stress.

- Foresight keeps you connected to what is real.

- Self-discipline is using the tools and a cushion of confidence.

- Courage shows your inner beauty.

- Grace is truth and beauty that shine through you.

I was advised, before going in front of TV cameras, to relax my mouth by relaxing my lips and then blowing through them. It makes a sound like a lawn mower engine trying to turn over. Look at yourself in the mirror and take a mental picture of your expression. Then, blow gently through relaxed lips and look at yourself again. What do you see?

> *'But I do know focusing on the exterior doesn't make me happy. If I want peace and serenity, it won't be reached by getting thinner or fatter.* [8] *Elle MacPherson, model*

- Food comes in at the mouth. Your mouth is sexy. Lips are for kissing, for laughing, smiling and opening the heart. A beautiful smile welcomes others into your world by putting them at ease. Pausing between bites, putting down the fork, smelling the aromas and just watching the others you're eating with, is beautiful.

- Calm gives space to sit on the edge of your moment and look into it. Find time to just 'be' with yourself. Go to your safe place and reaffirm your tools to connect with the feeling of balance. Feel it. It feels like a gentle flood of relief. Relaxation is beautiful.

- The next time you think about a great meal - let a whole world of possibilities open up. Seek a taste of something exotic. Trying new foods and new approaches to satisfying your appetite can be beautiful.

The reason for living is to be fully alive. Part of beauty is feeling beautiful. Following an intuitive lifestyle puts you on top of your game. You feel relaxed and beautiful, because you are.

Factoids

- Potato chips were invented in Saratoga Springs in 1853 by Native American chef, George Crum, in response to a patron who complained that his French fries were too thick. He thought he would rile the critical guest by giving him potatoes that could not be skewed with a fork, but it backfired when the guest loved the browned paper-thin potatoes! Now, potato chips are American's favorite snack food. A pound of potato chips costs two hundred times more than a pound of potatoes.[7]

- Although Europeans seem to love American trends, our oversized plates and supersized servings are not being imitated. The standard restaurant plate in Europe is 10". Here are some facts from Self Magazine:

  - Fries: UK of 5.5 oz. is 485 calories. US. super-size serving of 7oz. is 610 calories.

  - French croissant: 2 oz. is 215 calories. US croissant: 4 oz. is 430 calories.

  - UK steak: 8 oz. serving is 545 calories. US steak: 20 oz. serving is 1,360 calories.

  "Think With The Senses; Feel With The Mind"
  Venice, Italy Biennale 2007

Chapter 27 : Comfort Food for Chefs

Some food memories are emotional bookmarks we associate with home or contentment. These are commonly called, 'comfort food'. Comfort food memories are like time capsules. You mostly carry them as smells or tastes, like popcorn at the movies, chicken soup, homemade cookies, homemade meatloaf or leftover mac and cheese. Some are especially comforting, like getting a bowl of ice cream as part of a celebration, or Sunday morning pancakes.

Fill in the blanks: "My favorite comfort food is _____. It reminds me of_____." When you eat comfort food, you reconnect with a feeling of well-being from your past and bring it to the present.

Mentioning comfort food to dieters brings a negative response, if speaking of a forbidden pleasure. Since comfort means reassurance this seems wrong but notoriously, comfort foods have been labeled as diet derailers. Talking to intuitive eaters about comfort foods was, well it was comforting. They had clear memories of a taste and smell and often a memory or association to go with it.

When Chef Julia Child was asked what food she considered a guilty pleasure, she responded, *"I have never felt guilt over any pleasure that I have had."*[1] However, Julia Child also said, *"Moderation. Small helpings. Sample a little bit of everything. These are the secrets of happiness and good health."*[2] Aha, Julia Child was an intuitive eater.

For this book, I spoke with many professional chefs who agreed that great chefs cook and eat intuitively. Importantly, the definition of intuitive eating with our emphasis on the five senses, and the importance of holistic balance, totally resonated with these professional eaters.

Great chefs cook from the heart, using their senses to know what's good. My curiosity was piqued and much to my delight, I learned chefs have comfort foods just like you and me. Some delicious comfort food recipes from these chefs are included in this chapter to celebrate the variety of foods from around the world.

In my search, I met Antoinette Bruno, CEO and Editor-In-Chief of www.StarChefs.com, "the magazine for culinary insiders." The site reaches far into the world of eating. For example, it lists restaurant jobs, introduces new chefs and lists fresh food markets in every state. The mission of StarChefs is to give chefs the tools they need to succeed. Among the many local food organizations StarChefs support is **www.farestart.org**, which is a culinary job training and placement program for the homeless and disadvantaged.

Antoinette writes about food for a living, searching for new trends in cooking and is very particular about where she eats. Using curiosity, she takes great care to choose wisely and won't eat the food when she doesn't know the quality of ingredients going into the preparation. When on the road and Antoinette learns her only choice is fast food, she doesn't eat. Instead, Antoinette goes to a local market and buys fruit to take the edge off of her hunger. This takes tenacity, courage and dignity.

Part of her job is to travel all over the world to meet chefs and taste their cooking. Antoinette travels 26 weeks a year tasting food, usually doing five tastings a day. One tasting is 4 dishes from a particular chef. Sometimes portions are in a tasting menu, which means they are smaller. But often, it's the full size portion, for example, 4 complete dinners or 4 complete pastries. Usually, she takes just two or three bites, which "sometimes is really hard." She uses prudence with self-discipline and foresight.

Antoinette is a professional eater with a beautiful figure that she works very hard to maintain using self-discipline with tenacity. She explained, *"Sometimes the tasting is really fantastic and I want to devour everything in front of me. I try not to let that happen, and I remember as those bites are going into my mouth, how much more I have to exercise the following morning because I ate them."* This is being honest with herself, and using foresight. She continues, *"I am completely aware of the relationship between the calories that go in my body and that I have to run them off afterwards."* Again, this is self-discipline with tenacity.

Like the rest of us, this CEO has times when she overeats. Antoinette told me the following *"terrible story"*, while laughing at the experience, clear that it was overeating, and that she enjoyed it completely. Aha, another intuitive hedonist! Ultimately, Antoinette spoke from a place of grace.

Here's the story: Antoinette and her editor, Katherine Martinelli, were in LA and had already done 6 tastings this day. Most of them were savory and substantial. At 10PM, their 7th tasting was at a burger joint. The tasting was four courses. They were given two, differently prepared, *"huge"* burgers, a side of fries, a plate of 10 different kinds of pickles and a dessert that was *"kind of like a 'ring ding'."* The plan was to take a bite of each burger and a taste of the sides.

"But," Antoinette says, *"The first burger comes out and it is just to die for. I mean, I can smell it. I can, its, its just, its seeping into my system and I cannot wait to take a bite of this burger."* She cuts the first burger in half and gives half to her editor. *"So I took my bite, and I was thinking about how great this burger was. I looked at Katherine, and she was already on her second bite. I picked mine back up and we both devoured the entire half."* The next burger came out of the kitchen, and again she cut it in half. It smelled equally delicious and they both devoured the second half. *"These burgers were so incredible. It was just so delicious."*..."*I didn't eat the French fries, I ate one fry and I just barely tasted the pickles, they were also on the burgers."* They ate the whole 'ring ding'. *"That was definitely a day of overeating. In general I try to keep the tasting to two or three bites."*

When on a tasting trip, Antoinette uses foresight to make her hour workout a priority, since she knows she'll be eating. Antoinette put in "extra time" after this burger feast. If morning meetings or conference calls are scheduled, she takes them while exercising on the elliptical trainer or treadmill. She doesn't abuse her body and is highly aware of the importance of balance. *"I like my body and I want to keep my body."*

When Antoinette returns home after these trips, for the first few days she has carrot, apple, beet, ginger juice for breakfast and a juice drink of celery, spinach, cucumber, tomato with some lemon juice for lunch. For dinner, she eats a regular meal. *"My body knows that it needs just liquid, and it needs to cleanse, and it needs to get rid of everything I ate."* Antoinette adds, if the trip was not abusive, she might just have juice in the morning when she gets home. She listens to her body.

Sometimes, when Antoinette returns home from a trip of tasting exotic or rich food, *"the only thing I want is a hamburger, but I won't do it. I will wait until I do my juice."* I asked, why not? *"Because I know that it's the last thing my body needs."* This is self-respect. Antoinette uses her mind to balance what she emotionally wants to eat, with what she knows is best for her whole self. She is intuitively aware of the important mind, body, emotion balance.

I asked Antoinette if she has food cravings. For Antoinette, it's about location and season. She's uniquely tuned into the seasons. *"When the first strawberries come out, I'm craving strawberries, and when the first pea shoots come out, I'm craving peas...It's almost like you smell it in the air."* She says locations remind her of specific foods, so when she's in specific places, she craves what's there.

We agree that America is a culture of bigness and talk about how common oversized food portions are. I asked her about portion control in the food service industry. Antoinette quickly points out a clear distinction between food service and fine dining. Portion size is not a problem in fine dining. Instead, *"it's a problem in the quick serve at the fast casual level of dining. It stems from a society looking for perceived value. They want to get the most for their dollar. I don't think it comes from somebody who prides themselves on food as something they enjoy vs something that they use for fuel."* People have bought into the advertising myth that bigger is better.

Without prodding from me Antoinette continued, *"There are still people who go to fine dining restaurants, who leave and say, 'Wow, I left hungry.' And I always want to challenge those people. You shouldn't leave full. You should feel satisfied."* As we continued speaking she said, *"People eat out of habit."*

We talked about new trends in cooking and eating, and I learned that more chefs are handcrafting their foods. It's called artisanal, which is when a chef makes everything from scratch such as cheese, pasta or bread. Additionally, more chefs are going back to the country of origin for inspiration for recipes. This means more ethnic foods. Yum.

A current cooking trend is a throwback to a long time ago, called "head to tail" cooking. This includes cooking the heart, tongue, liver, lungs and inside organs of the animal. These are nutritious and tasty.

Currently, many new serious chefs are starting out by setting up food stands in trucks; so keep your eyes open and enjoy the treat if any roll you way. Lastly, Antoinette mentioned that there is a new trend in creating unique cocktails. It's called mixology. We're in for a good time.

Antoinette reveals her favorite comfort food without hesitation, *"My mother makes the best crab cakes I've ever eaten in my life, naturally bringing back childhood and home memories."* She has even posted her mom's recipe on-line at **starchefs.com/features/crabcakes/html/**

Overall, the trend is moving towards connecting with our "source" so that we can eat intelligently and not abusively. It's intuitive.

It was great fun collecting these delicious and unique recipes from celebrity chefs. You'll notice that two are mac & cheese, submitted by Chef Simon & Chef Ineke, and both have the familiar warm comforting effect. Both Chef Leal & Chef Ineke submitted recipes for chicken soup. The chicken soups are continents apart, yet both delicious and nurturing. Chicken soup is a universal comfort food. It's great a have a quart stashed away in the freezer for when you or someone you love needs comforting.

Recipes:

Kerry Simon

Celebrity Chef Kerry Simon is considered a visionary. He loves pure simple flavors of American cooking. This past year he opened Cat House at the Luxor Hotel and Simon at the Palms Casino Resort in Las Vegas. He has appeared on Iron Chef America, challenging and defeating Cat Cora in Battle: Hamburger. I was surprised when Chef Simon told me his favorite comfort food was Macaroni & Cheese. However, once I cooked his recipe, there was no doubt in my mind that it is the most decadent and divine mac & cheese ever!

The truffle oil makes this especially comforting. I served it with a simple green salad and we all felt the meal was perfect.

Truffle Macaroni & Cheese

2 cups heavy cream

1 3/4 cups shredded Monterey and sharp cheddar. (7/8ths cup ea) Set aside 1/4 cup of the mixture.

Kosher salt

Ground black pepper

2 tablespoons white truffle oil

3 cups cooked elbow macaroni noodles

1/4 cup grated Parmesan cheese

1/8th cup Japanese (panko bread) breadcrumbs

-Preheat oven to 350°F.

-Bring cream to a simmer and whisk in 1-1/2 cups grated cheese mixture.

-Season with salt, pepper, and truffle oil.

-Mix in cooked pasta.

-Pour into a large casserole or individual, 4-ounce casseroles or ramekins.

-Top with mixture of the Parmesan cheese, breadcrumbs and the remaining 1/4 cup of the cheese mixture

-Bake for 12 minutes, until golden brown and hot all the way through.

- Optional: You can place it under the broiler and cook until golden brown.

Serves 4 as a generous main course.

Marc Murphy

Celebrity Chef Marc Murphy, who currently has three stylish, and very popular restaurants in NYC, Landmarc (Tribecca), Ditch Plains, and Landmarc (at The Time Warner Center) finds comfort in the delicious flavors of this simple-to-make and mouth-watering pasta dish.

Orecchiette All Norcina

2 tablespoons olive oil

1 pound Italian pork sausage (preferably without fennel seeds), casing removed, crumbled

2 cloves garlic, thinly sliced

2 cups heavy cream

1/2 cup grated Parmesan cheese

2 teaspoons chopped rosemary

Kosher salt

freshly ground black pepper

1 pound orecchiette

- Bring one gallon of water to boil.   Add 2 tablespoons salt. Add pasta and cook 10 to 12 minutes.

 - Meanwhile, heat olive oil in a large saute pan over medium heat. Add sausage and sauté until cooked through, about 8 minutes.

- Add garlic and cook 1 minute.

- Add cream and rosemary and bring to a boil.

- Add drained pasta to pan and cook for 5 minutes.

- Add Parmesan and cook for 3 more minutes, tossing frequently.

- Season to taste with salt and pepper and serve.

6 servings (8 cups)

Joey Reynolds

Talk show host and celebrity chef, Joey Reynolds, "tells it like it is" on NYNBC five nights a week and everybody is listening. Often outrageous, always kind, Joey intuitively gets right to what's real. Well, his favorite comfort food is real! This lite cheesecake was created when, as a single dad, Joey had to take something to a picnic. He *"threw together"* this silky cheesecake using leftovers that were in his fridge, and it turned out to be a super star. Sold commercially for years, all proceeds went to charity. Just like Joey, this cheese cake is smooth and sweet without being heavy, and ultimately, a superstar comfort food that hits the spot. Delicious, easy to make and impressive to serve, you can understand how this is Joey's choice.

Lite Cheesecake

Crust:

In a Cuisinart mix:

2 packs of graham crackers

1 stick of butter, melted

2 tablespoons sweetener

Line springform pan with the crust. You can spread it around with a spoon and press it into corners gently with your finger tips.

Filling:

4 (8 ounce) bars fat free cream cheese

2 cups sugar or comparable stevia

4 eggs

2 limes

In a Cuisinart

Put in cream cheese, whip until creamy.

Add 2 cups sugar.

Squeeze in 1 lime.

Add 1 egg at a time.

Pour custard into crusted pan.

Bake for 40 minutes at 350°F.

Cool pan for 10 minutes.

Topping:

Stir together

1 Breakstone 8 ounce sour cream

4 tablespoons sweetener

1 tablespoon pure almond extract

Cover custard with this after it has cooled.

Place back in the oven for 10 minutes.

Refrigerate and enjoy the next day....

*All of the sweetening and fat ingredients can be substituted to diet.

Joyce Trimper

Chef Joyce Trimper is Antoinette Bruno's Mom's recipe. She's from Ocean City, MD The most important element to making crab cakes or any crab dish is not to overpower the delicate taste of blue crab. Let the crab flavor be dominant. Always use the best crabmeat you can find and make sure it's fresh.

Mom's Crab Cakes

1 pound jumbo lump crabmeat

I egg beaten

3 tablespoons mayonnaise

1 tablespoon dry mustard

1/2 bunch parsley, minced

7 saltine cracker halves, crushed

Light canola oil, for frying

Dash of salt and cayenne pepper

Mix all wet ingredients except the crabmeat. Then mix in the dry ingredients. Season with a dash of salt and cayenne pepper.

Fold in crabmeat last, being careful not to break apart the lumps. Delicately mold 5 large crab cakes.

Deep fry in light canola oil until golden brown.

CakesYield: 5 large crab cakes

Edgar Leal

Celebrity Chef Edgar Leal is co-host of the cooking show for CASA club TV (MGM Latin America), which airs all over South America. Cacao, his restaurant in Coral Gables, was named one of America's top 10 restaurants by Zagat. Now, Edgar is opening a new and very beautiful restaurant called Mohedano in La Castellana in Caracas, Venezuela.

Edgar invited me into his home to talk about comfort foods and cooking. For this mega-talented chef, the restaurant business is about being with friends. His wife Mariana, also a chef, works with him and every night, his restaurant is a celebration of the joys of cooking and eating together. That same warm, unique and embracing energy is clearly the taste of Venezuelan chicken soup, Edgar's comfort food. This recipe was easy to make, nourishing, incredibly delicious and freezes well.

Venezuelan Chicken Chupe

1 chicken weighing 3pounds

3 quarts water

The white part of 1 leek diced

1 tablespoon of olive oil

1 big onion diced

1 red pepper diced

1 1/2 cups of fresh corn

2 cups of diced potato

1 cup of medium diced carrots

6 garlic cloves minced

1 tablespoon of salt

1/2 teaspoon of ground white pepper

12 asparagus spears blanched cut each 1/2 inch long pieces

4 tablespoons of cilantro chopped

1 teaspoon of Tabasco sauce

2 cups of fresh white cheese cut in medium dices (I used Seaside English Cheddar)

1 cup of milk

1/2 cup of heavy cream

- Skin the chicken and place in a pot. Add the water and bring to a boil. Once it boils, turn it down to simmer and let it cook for 30 minutes.

- Take the chicken (strain) after those 30 minutes and let it cool down.

- Turn off the pot.

- Put a frying pan on medium heat. Add the oil, once the oil is hot put in the onions and the garlic to caramelize. Stir around with a wooden spoon. Add the red peppers and the leeks. Once all the ingredient start to turn caramel color, put this mixture into the chicken stock.
- Turn the pot back on, and put in the potatoes, the corn and the carrots. Once it boils. turn it down to simmer. Let it cook for 25 minutes.
- Dice the chicken.
- Add the asparagus, chicken, milk, heavy cream, Tabasco, cilantro salt, and pepper.
- Bring soup back to boiling; serve it in the bowls ready to eat.
- In the serving bowl add the diced cheese.

Serves 6 as a generous main course.

Chef Leal also shared the recipe below because it is a favorite one from his Caocao restaurant. You will need to make rice and a vegetable in advance because this cooks for just 10 minutes. It's delicious.

Margaritan Island style Seafood

1 full pound mussels

1 full pound shrimps

1 full pound squid

2 full pounds whole peeled tomatoes, diced

1/2 of cup of olive oil

1 big red onion diced

1 big red or yellow pepper diced

3 ajies Dulce (sweet peppers) diced

4 garlic cloves minced

4 Tablespoons of thinly cut cilantro

salt and pepper

- Clean all the Seafood.

- In a pot sauté with the olive oil, the onions, the peppers, the ajies and the   garlic.

- Add all the seafood and tomatoes and let it cook for 10 minutes

- Add the cilantro

- Once it's ready, serve with white rice and vegetables.

Serves 4.

Dorian Bergen

Dorian Bergen began baking in the 1970s at Ananda East Bakery, the largest natural foods bakery on the East Coast at that time. Over a ten year period, she cooked for hundreds of people at the Findhorn Community in Scotland. Additionally, Dorian has been a cook at the Rudolf Steiner School in New York City. This chef's recipes evolve intuitively. Dorian is passionate about serving delicious nourishing food and slips vegetables into meals without people noticing. This recipe is her family comfort food and can be served as a vegetable or for dessert. Children of all ages love this delicious treat.

Pumpkin Pie

29 oz pumpkin pulp (1 large can or 2 small ones) or 1 medium pumpkin

4 eggs

2 teaspoons cinnamon

1 teaspoon ground ginger

1/4 teaspoon ground cloves

1/2 teaspoon salt

1/2 teaspoon vanilla (powered or extract)

1/2 cup raw sugar (or any granulated sugar or sugar substitute)

1/2 cup maple syrup

12 oz milk (can be substituted with soy or almond milk)

9 inch pie crust or a graham cracker crust for special occasions

2-3 custard cups (These are to be used for any extra pumpkin mixture.)

Preheat oven to 425°F.

Use a Cuisinart or electric blender. The ingredients fit exactly into a Cuisinart.

*It is important to add the milk a little at a time at the end or the mix will spill over the edge

- Blend together the pumpkin pulp, eggs, cinnamon, ginger, cloves, salt, vanilla, raw sugar and maple syrup. Add the milk last.

-Pour the fully blended mixture into the pie crust. Pour any extra mixture into custard cups.

- Bake at 425°F for 20 minutes. Reduce the heat to 375°F and bake for an additional 55-65 minutes.

- Stick a sharp knife or cake tester into the center.

When done, the knife will come out clean. The custards can be removed first. This pie is moist so an extra 10 minutes will be fine. You can also let it cool in the oven when done.

Maria Canora

Personal Chef Maria Canora comes from a respected lineage of Italian chefs and her comfort food is as rich and noble as one could want for real comfort. Since it cooks for several hours without too much attention, and freezes well, this can be made in advance and then enjoyed at leisure. This meat sauce is served on cooked pasta. It is perfect for company and also great for kids.

Besides being a personal chef for families, Maria is on a mission to educate children about health and nutrition. She has won awards for her work teaching schools to make better quality lunches. Additionally, Maria created interactive after school workshops for inner city elementary children called the "Guess What Club" that benefits children and their parents. This recipe is her family favorite.

Salsa alla Bolognese

1/4 lb. ground veal

1/4 lb. ground beef

1/4 lb. ground pork

1 large white onion

1 carrot

1 stalk celery

2-3 cloves garlic

1 teaspoon basil

1/2 teaspoon thyme

1 teaspoon oregano

1/2 cup extra virgin olive oil

1/2 glass red wine

2 cups fresh chopped tomatoes

2 teaspoons tomato paste

1/2 teaspoon fresh ground nutmeg

salt and pepper to taste

grated Parmesan cheese (optional)

Preparation:
- Finely chop carrot, celery, and onion.
- Heat olive oil in heavy saucepot; add sosfritto (vegetable mixture).
- Caramelize mixture just until tender and light brown color is extracted,
- Add garlic and cook 5 minutes more.
- Add ground meats and cook until meats are very browned and stick to bottom of pot.
- Add wine and deglaze by scraping bottom of pot as wine is evaporating.
- Add tomato paste, chopped tomatoes, nutmeg, spices, salt and pepper.
- Let cook for 1 to 2 hours.

Serves 6 people.

To serve: Toss a small amount with the pasta and then place a small amount on top of the pasta.

Ciro

The man behind the popular global chain, Ciro's Pomodoro restaurants, is also a very busy humanitarian, a film producer, and privately, an angel. He has been working since he was 12 years old, and now regularly shakes hands with celebrities and dignitaries worldwide. In fact, it is typical for Ciro to be active on 3 different continents in one week. At the same time, this very private and spiritual person is always willing to help a friend. He is kind, humble, gracious, and very connected.

Ciro's favorite comfort food is classically elegant, tasty, health oriented, simple to make, and leaves you feeling satisfied. It reflects the man.

Fusilli Alla Checca

The sauce can be prepared while the pasta is cooking.

6 ounces Fusilli pasta

7 ounces fresh chopped tomato (the san Marzano

Tomato)

4 tablespoons extra virgin olive oil

1 fresh garlic clove chopped very small

4 fresh basil leaves (leave 2 whole and chop 2)

salt and paper to taste

Cooking the pasta:

-Put 1-1/2 quarts of water in pot with 2 teaspoons of salt and bring to a boil. Add the pasta.

-Cook for 6 minutes if you like it firm, or cook for 8 minutes.

Sauce:

-Put 2 teaspoon of extra virgin olive oil in a frying pan

-Add the chopped garlic and stir. As soon the garlic start turning golden,

-Add in the fresh tomatoes and 2 fresh basil leaves.

-Add the salt and pepper.

-Let it cook for 3 minutes.

Finishing:

-Drain the pasta and add to the sauce.

-Saute the pasta and the sauce together briefly.

-Put it on the plate and top with 2 teaspoon of extra virgin olive oil and chopped fresh basil.

This serves one person as a main course.

Annette Sym

Annette Sym, a best-selling cookbook author in Australia. She weighed 183 pounds when just 13 years old, and it was at that time she turned to traditional dieting. Ultimately, she learned that it didn't work. In 1992, Annette decided to take control of her life by eating what made sense to her intuitively.

I met Annette when she was touring this country to promote "Symply Too Good to Be True" which has tasty, low-fat, healthy recipes that she created for maintaining her healthy weight. About this comfort food dessert, Annette wrote: *"The old Annette who once weighed 220lbs would eat desserts all the time but wouldn't do them the healthy way and it showed ... she was overweight and unhealthy and not very proud of herself. Having lost over 70lbs which took me 20 months to lose, I found that doing desserts like the Fruit and Nut Cobbler helped support me along the way to my goal weight. Now after being in my healthy weight range for over 17 years, this is still one of my all time favourites."*

Annette likes to eat this warm and enjoys the crunchy top. It gives her peace of mind knowing this is "guilt free and healthy for you."

Fruit 'n' Nut Cobbler

Filling

2lb green apples

1/4 cup water

2 teaspoons sugar

1 x 14 1/2 oz can peaches in natural juice drained

Topping

1 1/2 cups Special K® cereal

1/2 cup self-rising flour

1/4 cup rolled oats

1/3 cup brown sugar

1/4 teaspoon cinnamon

1/4 cup pecan nuts

2 tablespoons light margarine melted (Promise®)

1 teaspoon no-fat milk

Preheat oven to 350°F (180°C)

To make filling:

-Peel and cut apples into quarters.

-Remove core then cut each quarter into 3 slices (4 for very large apples).

-Place in a large microwave dish with 1/4 cup water and sugar.

-Microwave on high for 6 minutes for 1200 watt microwave or 8 minutes for lower watt microwaves or until apple is just cooked but still firm.

-Drain apples and peaches then spread over the base of a casserole or small lasagne dish.

-Combine fruits together.

To make topping:

-In a medium size mixing bowl crush Special K using either potato masher or your fist.

-Add flour, oats, sugar and cinnamon.

-Chop pecan nuts into small pieces then add to bowl and combine well.

-Add melted margarine to milk then pour into bowl and combine with dry ingredients. You may find using your hand to combine mixture works best.

-Sprinkle mixture over top of fruit.

-Bake 30 minutes or until browned.

This serves 8. Not suitable to be frozen.

Variations:

Replace suggested fruit with any fruit of your choice or replace Special K with bran flakes or corn flakes.

Dietician's tip:

Peaches and apples have a low Glycemic Index and are an ideal dessert for people with diabetes.

Nutritional Information
Per Serve

Calories	167	Sugar	17.2g

Fat Total	4.2g	Fiber	2.3g
Saturated	0.5g	Protein	3.3g
Sodium	132mg	GI Rating	Medium
Carbs	29.5g		

Michael Psilakis

Celebrity Chef Michael Psilakis believes *"comfort food should allow you to journey back into fond memories."* He is an artist and poet in the kitchen, as well as with words. As we spoke about the delicious recipe for this book, he mentioned memories of his mother cooking. Chef Psilakis said, comfort food should be like a *"seed that blooms into a flower that places you in a moment that brings a smile to your face."*

Chef Psilakis identifies with his Greek heritage and fuses that style of cooking with his American roots to create unforgettable dishes at two of his NYC restaurants, Anthos and Kefi. Anthos is the only Greek restaurant in the USA to have received a prestigious Michelin star rating. Kefi serves casual comfort foods. Both reflect Chef Psilakis' respect for food and his cooking artistry.

Tsoutsoukakia (Meatballs, Roasted Garlic, Olives, Tomato)

For the meatballs:

1/2 lb ground pork

1/2 lb ground lamb

1/4 ground beef

1 onion chopped

4 garlic cloves chopped

6 garlic cloves roasted and pureed

2 tbs. chopped fresh dill

2 tbs. chopped fresh parsley

Salt & pepper to taste

1 tbs. Dijon mustard smooth

8 slices of white bread crust removed

1 cup milk

Flour

extra virgin olive oil

For the Sauce:

3 tbs. extra virgin olive oil

6 pieces of raw garlic

1 large onion, chopped

1/2 cup red wine

2 cups beef and chicken broth

2, 16 oz. cans Italian plum tomatoes in sauce

2 fresh bay leaves

To Garnish:

1/2 cup of tsakistes olives, pitted and cut in half

1/2 cup thassos or kalamata olives, pitted and cut in half

16 whole roasted garlic cloves, peeled

Fresh parsley, dill, mint, chopped

dried Greek oregano

Serves 4-6

Yield 6 meatballs each about the size of golf balls.

For the Sauce:

-Place oil in pan over medium heat,

-Sauté garlic and onions until golden brown.

-Deglaze with red wine.

-Reduce until almost dry.

-Add stocks and tomatoes crushed by hand a bit,

-Add bay leaf and simmer.

For the Meatballs:

-Put everything in a mixing bowl with the exception of the bread and milk.

-In a separate bowl, soak bread in milk until saturated and soft.

-Remove bread from milk, squeezing to drain off extra milk.

-Add to meat mixture and mix well to thoroughly incorporate.

-Form football shaped meatballs (about 1 1/2 " long).

-Dredge with flour, and pan-fry in until brown on all sides,

-Then transfer to a paper towel.

-Once all meatballs have been browned, add them to the pot with the tomato sauce and ----Braise for an hour.

-Season with salt and pepper.

Right before serving, add the olives, roasted garlic cloves, fresh herbs and dried Greek Oregano to the meatball/tomato mixture. Stir to combine and serve.

Patrick Lapaire

Award-winning Chef Patrick Lapaire does a serious swimming workout every morning before he goes to work at The Alexander Hotel and Shula's Steakhouse in Miami. Chef LaPaire is very health oriented, and his comfort food is an amazing salad. Born in Switzerland, his inspiration comes from summers spent at his grandparent's bucolic home in the mountains, where they grew everything the family ate. He especially remembers the smell and taste of berries warmed by sunlight. This salad for one, is named for his daughter, Alexandra.

Alexandra Spring Salad with Lobster medallions, Grilled Shrimp & Fig Balsamic Bouquet

3 oz organic mixed baby greens leaves

6 oz lobster tails

2 jumbo shrimps

2 or 3 blackberries, blueberry, raspberries and strawberries

5 each dry raisins

1/2 fresh mango

1/4 apple & pear

1 fl/oz fig balsamic bouquet

2 1/2 fl/oz extra virgin olive oil

Feta cheese

Preparation:

-Cook the lobster in boiling water with a pinch of salt and 1 lemon

-Split the lobster tail in half, the take meat out of the shell. Slice the tail into identical round pieces,

-Brush the 2 shrimp with paprika and grill.

-Place a 12 inch red tomato & basil tortilla chip in a fryer for 3 minutes so that it forms the shape of the mesh basket. This will be the 'bowl' for the salad.

-In large bowl toss the mixed greens salad with the fig bouquet & extra virgin olive oil

-Put the mixed salad in the tortilla bowl

All of the other ingredients are placed on top of the greens but not mixed.

-top with all the berries and the raisins

-shred the apple & pear into little sticks (mandolin)

-arrange the lobster & shrimp.

-slice the mango thin and fan it out

-cut sticks of feta cheese and place on top of greens

-drizzle the rest of the oil & fig bouquet on top

Served with any kind of fresh fruit juice.

"I like Apple juice from La Motta or Cranberry Bon appétit!"
Patrick Lapaire

Richard O'Connell

Chef Richard O'Connell is executive chef at The Groucho Club in London. This private club is named after Groucho Marx because of his famous remark that he would "not wish to join any club that would have him as a member". Groucho members are from the worlds of entertainment, fashion, the arts, and media. They are visually-oriented and discriminating. Chef O'Connell knows how to please this tough crowd. The following recipe, created by Chef O'Connell, is a favorite of the members of The Groucho Club. It is beautiful to look at and full of flavor.

Carpaccio of Watermelon / feta cheese/ walnut / bean & chicory salad

For the melon:

Cut the melon into 4 and peel the one you want to use.

Place on the slicing machine & lay out neatly on the plate

Or slice really thin with a knife

For the cheese:

Place 4 ounces of cheese on a sheet of plastic wrap.

Add another sheet on top and roll with a rolling pin to get a sheet of cheese

Cut with a ring cutter and leave aside

For the salad:

Blanch and cut the beans into thin strips (about 7)

Wash & cut chicory into thin strips

Caramelise the walnuts with some sugar

Make a basic vinaigrette (3 parts oil to 1 part vinegar – Splash of lemon)

To Finish:

Brush the melon with the dressing

Add the cheese in the centre

Mix all salad and season & dress

Assemble on the cheese with some pea shoots

Add a couple of drops of balsamic reduction (available at most food supermarkets)

Eat & enjoy.

Chef O'Connell's personal comfort food, after a tough night, is a posh croque monsieur, which is delicious.

Posh Croque Monsieur

1 x loaf of brioche bread (brioche is a light French bread rich in butter and eggs, if unavailable substitute your favorite bread)

2-3 slices of good Parma ham or any other cured ham that you like

1 poached egg

2 good slices of your favorite cheese – cheddar – gruyere – brie

some nice mixed salad leaves

Preparation:

-Slice the brioche twice to give you 2 thick slices

-Butter them , then add the cheese onto one side and the ham on the other side.

-Place on a tray and then under the grill, grill until the cheese is melted and the bread toasted.

-Put them together to make a sandwich. Then grill them until both sides are golden brown.

-*"If you want to you can remove the crusts, but I say don't bother."*

Serve this with a runny poached egg on top and some dressed salad on the side.

Ineke

Ineke is the Chef at Indomania, a Dutch-Indonesian restaurant in Miami Beach. She and her husband are also the owners, and this small, stylish, streamlined environment is a gem. The hospitality and food feel homey even if one has never been to Indonesia. Smells and colors are both exotic and comforting. Chef Ineke's comfort food is the light and satisfying Indonesian Chicken soup recipe below. Unfortunately, I had difficulty finding several of the ingredients for this soothing chicken soup that bursts with flavor. **templeofthai.com/cooking/ingredients.php** was a helpful site for ingredients.

Soto Ayam Indonesian Chicken Soup

The Broth:

2 1/2 quarts of water

1 whole chicken or 5 full pieces of chicken

1 teaspoon of salt

Simmer for one hour.

Skim off foam.

The Spice Mix:

1 red onion
5 garlic cloves
5 candlenuts or macadamia nuts
1 inch ginger root

Mix these in a blender until a smooth paste then,

Fry in 2 teaspoons of oil.

Add to above:

1 teaspoon turmeric

2 teaspoons coriander powder
2 teaspoons galangal powder (ginger mixed with lemon juice)
5 lime leaves (possibly hard to find, can substitute lemon thyme, or sweet basil)
5 Daun Salam leaves (substitute is bay leaves)
1 lemongrass stick
salt and pepper

Next:
Strain the chicken broth and shred the white meat.
Add the spice mix to the broth and
Simmer for 15 minutes.
Add the shredded chicken

Serve with:
Glass noodles (a 2 ounce package)
1 tablespoon bean sprouts (per person)
1/2 hard boiled egg, chopped (per person)
1 teaspoon fried shallots and friend scallions (per person)
a slice of lemon
This soup serves 6 people.

Additionally, Chef Ineke shared a wonderful comfort food her family, especially the children, love. When I first looked at this pasta recipe, I wondered if it would appeal to Americans like myself.

What a great surprise to discover it is easy to prepare, delicious, light, and comforting. The sauce can be made in advance. Also, if you make extra, it's good reheated. This can easily become a family favorite. It's a lot like mac & cheese.

Pasta with Blue Cheese Sauce

10 ounce turkey breast

2 tablespoons butter

2 tablespoons oil (I used light olive oil)

1 cup sour cream

1 cup gorgonzola cheese (cut into cubes)

milk or water (optional)

1 pound penne pasta

-Put on water to boil for the pasta.

-Cut turkey breast into small bite sized pieces. Saute over medium heat in   the   butter and oil.

-Add the sour cream and the gorgonzola cheese and stir a few times. If   sauce is too thick, milk or water may be added. (I did not find this necessary.)

-Cook the pasta.

-Toss the pasta with sauce and serve.

This generously serves 4 as a main course.

Allan Wyse

Personal Chef Allan Wyse is a chef to stars such as Jon Bon Jovi, Billy Joel, Tyra Banks, Kim Cattrall and Fran Dresher. Born in Canada to 'hippy" parents, Allan naturally sees outside the box and feels in sync with nature. He cooks following his intuition and this empowering balance of nature and intuition permeates his life. He finds comfort in nature, and for *Am I Really Hungry?*, Allan created four salads using the bounty of each season that he calls, "Man-Salads". These are beautiful to look at, satisfying and delicious.

"Man Salads" designed for the seasons

Winter

Duck breast with roasted buttercup squash, toasted walnuts, blood orange, frisee lettuce, goat cheese, and finished with a pomegranate thyme vinaigrette.

1 large duck breast

1 buttercup squash (medium dice)

1 blood orange (segmented)

1/2 cup walnuts (toasted)

3 oz goat cheese

2 heads frisse lettuce (cleaned)

1 pomegranate (juiced)

3 sprigs fresh thyme

3 tablespoons grape seed oil (or other neutral oil)

1 tablespoon red wine vinegar

salt and pepper to taste

- First make the vinaigrette with the grape seed oil, red wine vinegar, 1 tablespoon of pomegranate juice, thyme leaves, a touch of water, and salt/pepper.

- Preheat oven to 400. Season duck breast with salt, and sear fat side down on a cast iron pan (or other heavy bottomed sauté pan) until very golden and crisp. Then place the duck breast in oven for 5 minutes or until it's cooked to medium. Allow the duck to rest for 20 minutes.

- Toss the diced squash lightly in oil, and salt, then place in the oven until tender and golden (approx 15 min). Let the squash cool.

- To finish toss the frisee, walnuts, goat cheese, blood orange segments, squash, and mix them with the vinaigrette. Then slice the duck breast very thin, and place on top of the salad.

Serves 2 – 4

Spring

Organic chicken breast with grilled spring asparagus, scallion, wild greens, crusty bread, Moncheago cheese chunks, and topped with a creamy lemon yogurt chive dressing.

2 organic chicken breasts

1 bunch asparagus (ends trimmed)

1 bunch scallion (washed)

8 oz wild greens (washed and dried)

baguette (or other crusty French bread)

4 oz Moncheago cheese (rough chunks)

1/4 cup pressed Greek yogurt

1 tablespoon olive oil

1 teaspoon lemon juice

fresh chives (minced)

salt/pepper to taste

- Fire up the grill to high heat.

- Make the creamy dressing. In a bowl whisk together the Greek yogurt, olive oil, chopped chives, and lemon juice (salt and pepper to taste).

- Season the chicken breast, asparagus, and scallion with salt/pepper/oil, and grill. Allow the chicken breast, and the veggies to rest. Slice the baguette into 1/2 rounds then grill until toasty and crispy.

- To finish put all ingredients together with the dressing, add salt and pepper if needed.

Serves 2 - 4

Summer

Heirloom tomatoes, creamy Boratta cheese, broiled shrimp, fresh basil, fennel, olive oil croutons, topped with a warm onion, and prosciutto vinaigrette.

8 oz heirloom tomatoes (mixed colors, and sizes)

4 oz Borrata cheese (or fresh mozzarella)

6 large shrimp (not peeled)

1 tablespoon paprika

1/2 bunch fresh basil

1 Fennel bulb

1 tablespoon lemon juice

crusty French bread

1/4 cup olive oil

1/2 cup Spanish onion (minced)

3 oz prosciutto

1 tablespoon sherry vinegar

salt/pepper

- Place the oven to broil.

- Season shrimp with salt/pepper/oil/paprika, and place under broiler for 2/3 minutes or until cooked through. Allow the shrimp to cool, and then peel them.

- Cut bread into 1/2 dice toss with salt. Then broil on the same vessel as the shrimp as to soak-up all the oil, and then toast until brown and crispy.

- Next make the warm vinaigrette. In a sauté pan on low heat add oil, onions, and cook them until they caramelized. Then remove the onions, and crisp up the prosciutto in the same pan. Add back the onions, the sherry vinegar, and salt and pepper (keep warm).

- Cut up the tomatoes into various shapes, and sizes then season with salt, and pepper.

- Slice the fennel very thin, and toss with lemon juice.

- To finish toss all ingredients together put on a platter, and spoon on the warm vinaigrette

Serves 2 – 4

Fall

"Vegetarian" salad with fingerling potatoes, chanterelles, roasted beets, crisp pear, green beans, lentils, watercress, and a shallot, grainy mustard dressing.

8 oz Fingerling potatoes

1/2 cup French green lentils

6 oz chanterelle mushrooms (brushed clean)

2 beets (medium size)

pear (firm, and crisp)

green beans

1 bunch watercress (cleaned)

1 tablespoon white wine vinegar

1 shallot (minced)

1 tablespoon grainy mustard

3 tablespoons olive oil

salt/pepper

- Preheat oven to 400°v.

- Season the beets with salt/pepper/oil then wrap each of them in aluminum foil, and place in the oven for 1 hour.   Let them cool, and then peel.

- Now make your dressing by adding the white wine vinegar, and a pinch of salt to the shallots for 15 minutes, then add the oil, a touch of water, the grainy mustard, and then adjust for seasoning.

- Place the fingerling potatoes in a size appropriate pot, fill it with water to cover them by at least four inches, and then add salt. Cook for around 20 minutes or until just tender, drain, and chill them.

- Place lentils in a pot, and fill with water, add salt, and a touch of olive oil. Cook for 15-20 minutes until tender, drain them, and chill.

-Bring a medium size pot full of water to a boil, add salt (until the water tastes like the sea), plunge in the green beans for 1 minute remove and place in a bath of ice/water.

-Heat a sauté pan to very high heat, pour in a small amount of oil, and sear off the mushrooms being very careful to not crowd the pan. Season them with salt/pepper, and reserve.

- Dice the pear, cut the beets into wedges, slice the potatoes into rings, and half the green beans.

- To finish place all ingredients together into a bowl, toss in the dressing, and season with salt/pepper.

Serves 2 – 4

Zoila Merlin

In the mountain village of Tlapa de Comonfort, in Guerrerro, Mexico, there is a small restaurant that has been open 7 days a week, almost 365 days a year, for nearly 40 years. The chef, proprietor and heart is Zoila Merlin. She starts early in the morning making sauces and soups, and the place is packed from morning til night with happy, hungry eaters. A popular comfort recipe is called, "Tinga".

Tinga

2 chicken breasts

1 chicken bouillon cube (optional)

½ pound tomatoes (no seeds because they cause a sour taste)

1 small potato diced

1 white onion

3 cloves garlic

¼ cup extra virgin olive oil

1 small can chipotle sauce

1 pack of corn tostadas (best when they are not too fresh)

1 head romaine lettuce, chopped

1 8oz Mexican style cultured cream (can substitute sour cream)

1 sliced avocado

1 pack of fresh Mexican cheese (optional)

-Boil the chicken until tender. Reserve water.

-Shred the chicken and set aside.

-Chop the garlic, onion, and tomatoes

-Blend 1 cup of chicken broth with the bouillon cube and the chipotle sauce.

-Saute the garlic for 1 minute in the olive oil, add the onion for 1 minute, then add the tomatoes, potatoes and chipotle sauce mix.

-Saute for 10 minutes. Then add the chicken and turn off heat.

-Put tostadas on plates. Place the chicken / vegetable mixture on top of the tostadas.

-Then top with lettuce, cheese and sour cream.

-Finish with slices of avocado on top.

Serves 2.

While writing this book, I discovered many chefs are also humanitarians. Like Chef Kerry Simon, and Dorian Bergen, Chef Galen Sampson is one.

Galen Sampson

Modest, discreet and hard working, Galen and his wife and partner, Bridget, have The Dogwood restaurant, which is a gem in Hampden section of Baltimore City. The food is locally grown whenever possible, so the menu always changes. Meals are beautifully presented and originally prepared, and delicious.

The Dogwood's social mission is to transform lives one plate at a time by providing training opportunity and paid employment to individuals who are transitioning from addiction, incarceration, homelessness, and/or underemployment.

Chef Galen and Bridget cook and eat intuitively. At their home, they grow herbs and vegetables. Chef Galen's comfort food recipe takes roast chicken to a new enjoyment level. In sync with his generosity of spirit, Galen included tips to make sure you find this recipe comforting to the last bite.

Galen and Bridget's Baked Organic Citrus-y Chicken

Ingredients:
1 small organic whole chicken
organic olive oil
3 cloves garlic, minced
2 carrots

3 ribs of celery
1 medium yellow onion
. cup rosemary and thyme leaves, chopped
4 sprigs rosemary
4 sprigs thyme
. bunch parsley
(use home grown or organic herbs if possible)
2 tsp sea salt
1 tsp black pepper
1 tsp ground coriander
1 orange
2 lemon

1. Preheat the oven to 425°F.
2. Rinse chicken thoroughly inside and out, remove giblets, pat dry.
3. Rough chop the onions, celery, carrots (mire poix).
4. Juice the orange and lemons.
5. Rough chop rosemary, thyme, and parsley.

(Perform steps 6-8 on the back and on the back and breast side,
    using half the amount of herbs and garlic on each side.)

6. Rub the chicken generously with olive oil.
7. Rub with the garlic.
8. Cover the chicken with chopped herbs.
9. Pour the lemon and orange juice over the chicken.
10. Stuff the chicken with mire poix and with the juiced rinds of
    orange and lemon.
11. Sprinkle black pepper, coriander and salt on the chicken.
12. Tuck rosemary and thyme sprigs under legs and wings.
13. Place chicken, breast side down in roasting pan.
14. Cook at 425°F for 20 minutes.
15. Turn oven down to 350°F.
16. Cook for 55 to 70 minutes, until internal temperature on thigh is
    165 F.
17. Allow bird to rest 10-15 minutes before carving.

Tips from Chef Galen:

- Use the two-stage method (Roast it fast. Cook it slow.) to get crisp skin and moist,tender insides. The two-stage method starts off at high heat (425°F) for 20 minutes.

- We then reduce the temperature to 350°F until done. Of course, the oven temperature does not go from 425°F to 350°F immediately, so the skin continues to crisp.

- We ease up on the cooking temperature to let the interior of the chicken slowly roast under the protection of its beautifully crisped skin.

Keep it moist! Cooking is strenuous as it boils the juices inside the chicken. This is why you need to let the bird rest: to let those juices slowly incorporate back into the flesh. If you cut into the chicken too soon, that moisture will run out onto your cutting board.

Bon Appetite!

Am I Really Hungry?

Chapter 28 : **The Emperor's New Diet**

There is a Hans Christian Anderson children's tale where all the people are under a lot of pressure, so they lie to themselves and to each other. The Emperor's New Clothes is about what happens when common sense meets fear and denial. In this story, adults are so humiliated and afraid of appearing unworthy, that they deny what their eyes see and what they absolutely know in their brain. They totally ignore their intuition.

The Emperor has hired con artists, who he believes are tailors, to fit him for a new outfit for a parade. They do this elaborately and precisely with a material they say is so precious that it can only be seen by those who are truly worthy. Everyone in the kingdom hears about this precious material that can only be seen by those who are worthy.

In fact, there is no material. But because the tailors 'see' it, the Emperor, fearing that he is unworthy, also praises the new suit even though he doesn't see or feel it. Members of the court deny their own eyes and agree that the suit looks fantastic.

As the Emperor parades through the streets expecting people to admire his new suit, they do... until a small child, watching with his parents, points at the naked Emperor and loudly says, "But he has nothing on!" and wham - common sense puts an end to the fear and denial. The moral is: If something doesn't look right or sound right to you, trust your intuition. It will be a huge relief and that's the naked truth.

Choices based on fear are often a form of self-denial. Eating in a way that doesn't relate to hunger because you're afraid of gaining weight, is self-denial because it's a disconnect from your intuition and your body.

Denying the natural balance of body, mind and heart creates a box of confusion, frustration and humiliation. When you decide to fine tune your senses and liberate yourself with the naked truth, you step right out of the box.

Depending on your tools and recognizing what you see, hear, taste, touch and smell, is the connection with your intuition that gives you an open mind and an empowering focus on healthy eating.

Grace is your intuitive connection with unique wisdom. Giving yourself a chance to succeed is common sense. When you're in sync with your senses, heart and mind, there is nothing to fear. You are grounded and alert.

By eating with dignity and patience, the right choice always feels easy. Instead of denial, use dignity to be in tune with your body and yourself.

The naked truth is that hunger is intensely personal, which means satisfying it is individual. It doesn't make sense to turn eating choices over to anyone. Certainly it makes sense to use curiosity to learn from others, but equally, you have to be clearly in tune with yourself. Use prudence to compare eating options, and dignity with patience to keep a flexible open mind. It makes sense to treat yourself with respect.

When open to the truth and in sync with yourself, you're living intuitively. Use the personal compass of honesty. If something feels wrong, it is wrong. You may not know why, but may be sure that with patience, you'll discover a truth.

The foundation of self-protection is honoring yourself by using and trusting your 6 senses. The intuitive tools are an arsenal of insight custom-tailored to your values and priorities. Depend on them and the reward is genuine.

The naked truth is that eating is intuitive. We eat to give our body nourishment to boost and sustain life. When you strip yourself of plans, programs and regimens, unique natural hunger patterns, needs and ways to enhance and protect yourself when you eat, become clear.

Hunger can be emotional as well as physical. Everyday stuff happens that impacts appetites and needs. Each meal is a new experience to eat what your body needs to empower you now.

- Tune into changes in your body. Connect with courage and fine tune with tenacity. Fear and denial are so yesterday.

- Stay connected to your wish bone, back bone and funny bone. No matter what you are worried about today, it will change.

- Depend on the tools and 5 senses. They are a direct connect to your 6th sense and hold the key to being in sync with yourself.

- At any time, pull the trigger to tune in for perspective; connect with what you need and how you feel.

Intuition connects with naked truths about who you are and what deeply matters in your life. When you're in sync, all choices are easier. As you get into the habit of depending on the tools, you'll discover that you're pretty amazing.

The Intuitive Eaters Tool Chest

Curiosity is your inner child – the one who questions from a place of flexible innocence, the one who only knows change, and is drawn towards truth. It is your free spirit.

Prudence is balancing options – the tool to recognize there are choices. Prudence balances past eating experiences with present needs and keeps you aware of different perspectives.

Tenacity is commitment to yourself. It's inner drive that honors your life.

Dignity is an attitude of self-respect seen through your actions. Dignity is a quiet power that grows with use.

Determination is natural enthusiasm. It's an intuitive vitamin bringing energy to boost the connection to your intuitive voice. Determination always hooks up with other tools. It's empowering.

Patience is breathing space. Patience helps you change with life's surprises, and stay in sync with yourself. Patience works with your body, mind and heart equally. It is the source of the empowering intuitive 'pause' that lets everything realign, so you can be clear about what you're doing.

Foresight is intuitive self-defense. By staying connected with the present, your perspective stays clear about healthy eating choices for your body.

Self-Discipline is deeply honoring yourself, which sounds so obvious, but in our superficial world, is a tool we must work to use. It is the essence of respecting yourself. Self-discipline is your natural guide.

Courage is the tool that you can count on to live in harmony with your own nature. It's a source of strength to trust yourself. By depending on courage, you recognize opportunities to honor your body by what you eat.

Grace is another chance to succeed. It works with all of the tools enhance momentum. It's never too early or too late to forgive yourself and move forward to achieve eating goals.

Focus is the intuitive magnifying glass. It strengthens and magnifies the intuitive connection created by your tools.

Honesty is the intuitive compass that always points to the long term, satisfying direction when you make eating choices.

Look into your eyes in the mirror and make a commitment to yourself. Notice what you see, listen to your heart, connect with your values and you have already begun. Use intuition to shift from old mindsets that harbor fears or denial, and embrace the freedom of self-control. Keep a clear purpose in your mind when you choose what to eat. Sometimes you're hungry for food, but sometimes you're hungry for change.

The naked truth is, right now you may not be happy with your body. Right now, you may seek a quick fix. There is no quick fix, but there is a fix, and it's a safe private place inside of you. Pull the trigger and use your intuitive tools. Intuition is your personal trainer. Take advantage of it. The intuitive tools are equipment to get you in shape. They can feel pretty heavy in the beginning. But the weight stays off.

Intuitive eating is not a quick fix. It's the answer.

IntuEating Journal Example

My Eating Journal
www.IntuEating.com

Hunger
1 - not hungry
2 - social hunger only
3 - normal / neutral
4 - more than usual
5 - cravings / strong urge
6 - starving / eat now!

Feeling
1 - intuitive / self-control
2 - satisfied / at ease
3 - normal / neutral
4 - tired / bored
5 - lonely / sad
6 - stressed / anxious

Self-Control
1 - Intuitive / automatic control
2 - moderate control
3 - normal / neutral
4 - borderline
5 - slipping
6 - out of control

Tools
a) Foresight /self-defense
b) Patience /breathing room
c) Curiosity / my 5 senses and my mind
d) Prudence /my options
e) Tenacity /commitment to myself
f) Dignity /self-respect
g) Determination / follow through
h) Self-discipline / my intuition
i) Courage / my Lifeline
j) Grace / personal forgiveness

Date/Time					
My Hunger					
My Feelings					
Self-Control					
Tools I Used					
My Food Choices					
Location					
My Thoughts					

Citations

The links listed below can below can also be found at:
www.intueating.com/6th-sense-eating/references.html

Introduction

1 Carroll, Lewis (Charles Lutwidge Dodgson). 1861. Through The Looking Glass and What Alice Found There. London, New York: Macmillan and Co.

Chapter 1: Intuition

1 Cummings, Laura. 2003. The diet business: Banking on Failure. BBC News World Edition. **news.bbc.co.uk/2/hi/business/2725943.stm**

2 Cummings, Laura. 2003. The diet business: Banking on Failure. BBC News World Edition. **news.bbc.co.uk/2/hi/business/2725943.stm**

3 Lucas, George. 1977. Star Wars movie. 20th Century Fox.

4 Lucas, George. 1977. Star Wars movie. 20th Century Fox.

5 Brown, Harriet. 2006. Go With Your Gut. The New York Times. **nytimes.com/2006/02/20/opinion/20brown.html**

6 Carey, Benedict. 2009. Gut Feeling Often Aids IED Detection. The San Diego Union Tribune. **nytimes.com/2006/02/20/opinion/20brown.html**

7 Arden, Paul. 2003. It's Not How Good You Are, It's How Good You Want To Be. London. Phaidon Press Ltd

8 St. Augustine. **thinkexist.com/quotes/saint_augustine/3.html**

9 Fielding, Henry. 1707-1754. **thinkexist.com/quotes/henry_fielding/**

10 Sontag, Susan. 1944-2004. **brainyquote.com/quotes/quotes/s/susansonta122012.html**

11 Gauguin, Paul. 1848-1903. **thinkexist.com/quotation/i_shut_my_eyes_in_order_to_s ee/218611.html**

12 Kohlstadt, Ingrid, ed. 2009. Food and Nutrients in Disease Management. FL: CRC Press: Taylor and Francis Group,

Chapter 2: Intuitive Tools
1 Rowling, JK. 1965- .
brainyquote.com/quotes/quotes/j/jkrowlin178383.html

Chapter 6: Dignity
1 Hanh, Thich Nhat. 1926- .
brainyquote.com/quotes/authors/n/nhat_hanh.html

Chapter 7: Determination
1 Lorimer, George. 1867-1937.
thinkexist.com/quotation/youve_got_to_get_up_every_morn
ing_with/207601.html

Chapter 8: Patience
1 Wooden, John. 1910- .
thinkexist.com/quotes/John_Wooden/
2 The Amazing Banana.
scionofzion.com/banana.htm

Chapter 9: Foresight
1 Covey, Steven. 1932- .
thinkexist.com/quotes/stephen_r._covey/

Chapter 10: Self-Discipline
1 Emerson, Ralph Waldo. 1803-1882.
Self-reliance and Other Essays, 1993,Dover Publications, Inc.
New York

Chapter 11: Courage
1 Lewis, C.S. 1898-1963.
brainyquote.com/quotes/quotes/c/cslewis100842.html
2 Shakespeare, William. 1564-1616;
Macbeth, Act 1, Scene 7. enotes.com/shakespeare-
quotes/screw-your-courage-sticking-place.
3 Churchill, Winston. 1874-1965.
brainyquote.com/quotes/quotes/w/winstonchu161628.html

Chapter 13: Transformational Eating, The Shift
1 Cohen, Alan. 1954- .
brainyquote.com/quotes/quotes/a/alancohen188584.html
2 Dixit, Jay. Senior Editor. How to Reprogram Mental Eating
Habits for Physical Success. Psychology Today Magazine.
2008 July/August

Chapter 14: Hunger
1 Flemming, Paul, 1609-1640.
crywithme.com/usm470452.html?t=Quotes
2 Osho, "Rajneesh" Chandra Mohan Jain. 1931-1990. Institute
for Integrative Nutrition. 2009
3 Hippocrates. 467 BC- 370 BC
goodreads.com/quotes/show_tag?name=Medicine
4 Davis, Adelle. 1904-1974.
quotationspage.com/quotes/Adelle_Davis/
5 Ford, Henry. 1863-1947.
brainyquote.com/quotes/quotes/h/henryford122817.html
6 Gabriel, Jon. 2009. The Gabriel Method. Australia: Simon &
Schuster
7 Hunger Hormone Ghrelin Increases During Stress, May Have
Antidepressant   Effect. June 2008.
news-medical.net/news/2008/06.24.39395.aspx
8 Weil, Andrew, MD. 1942- .
thinkexist.com/quotation/pay-attention-to-your-body-the-
point-is-everybody/367743.html
9 Wade, Nicholas. 2005. Your Body Is Younger Than You
Think. The New York Times.
nytimes.com/2005/08/02/science/02cell.html?_r=1&pagewant
ed=print
10 McCord, Holly, RD. McVeigh, Gloria. Busted! 5 Major
Eating Mistakes. 2007. Prevention.com
search.prevention.com/vignette/pvn/search.jsp?num=20&re
quiredfields=pvsrch:1.pv_type:10&q=elisabetta%20Politi,
%20RD
11 Gabriel, Jon. 2009. The Gabriel Method. Australia: Simon&
Schuster

Chapter 15: Frustration
  1 Schuller, Robert J. 1926 -   .
  saidwhat.co.uk/quotes/favourite/robert_schuller
  2 Eliot, George. 1819-1880.
  brainyquote.com/quotes/authors/g/george_eliot_6.html
  3 Coolidge, Calvin. 1872-1933.
  quotationspage.com/quotes/Calvin_Coolidge/
  4 Markova, Dawna. Educator and Speaker.

Chapter 16: Understanding Change
  1 Cowper, William. 1731-1800.
  brainyquote.com/quotes/quotes/w/williamcow383185.html
  2 de Sales, St. Francis. 1567-1622.
  brainyquote.com/quotes/quotes/s/saintfranc193306.html
    3 Shakespeare, William. 1564.1616. "The Tempest"
  4 Pope, Alexander 1688-1744. An Essay On Criticism
  5 The Medical News from News-Medical.net, Anticipation of
  Laughter Reduces Levels of Stress Hormones. April 2008.
  news-medical.net/news/2008/04/08/37095.aspx
  6 Song, Sora. 2008. Five Stealth Forces In Weight Loss.
  Psychology Today,   July/August 2008
  7 Rooney, Mickey. 1920-   .
  quotationspage.com/quote/1627.html

Chapter 17: The Plan
  1 Blatner, Dawn Jackson, RD, LDN. 2008. The Flexitarian Diet:
  the mostly vegetarian way to lose weight, be healthier, prevent
  disease and add years to your life. McGraw-Hill

Chapter 18: The Mystery Tool – Grace
  1 Rae-Dupree, Janet. 2008. Can You Become a Creature of New
  Habits?. The New York Times.
  nytimes.com/2008/05/04/business/04unbox.html?_r=1&scp=
  1&sq=Can%20You%20become%20a%20creature%20of%
  20new%20habits?&st=cse
  2 ibid
  3 ibid

4 Anglier, Natalie. 2008. Mirrors Don't Lie. Mislead? Oh, Yes. The New York Times. **nytimes.com/2008/07/22/science/22angi.html?sq=The%20Mi rror,%20July%202008&st=cse&scp=1&pagewanted=print** 5 de Sales, St. Francis. 1567-1622. **brainyquote.com/quotes/authors/s/saint_francis_de_sales.ht ml** 6 Larson, Johathan. 1960-1996. Rent. "Seasons of Love". **majannmariedaneker.blogspot.com/2009/01/how-do-you-measure-year.html** 7 de Sales, St. Francis. 1567-1622. **brainyquote.com/quotes/quotes/s/saintfranc131350.html** 8 Rush University Medical Center. 2009. Health Information, Determining Your Ideal Weight. **rush.edu/rumc/page-1108048103230.html**

Chapter 19: Falling Off The Wagon

1 Burns, Robert. 1759-1796. **thinkexist.com/quotes/robert_burns/** 2 LeDoux, Joseph. Synaptic Self: How Our Brain Becomes Who We Are. 2002. New York. Viking Penguin Press. 3 Angier, Natalie. 2008. The Nose, an Emotional Time Machine. The New York Times. **nytimes.com/2008/08/05/science/05angier.html** 4 Leschak, Peter. 2002. Ghosts of the Fireground: Echos of the Great Peshtigo Fire and the Calling of a Wildland Fire. New York: HarperCollins Publishers Inc. 5 Loudon, John. 1985. Experiments in Truth. Parabola Winter Vol. 10:4. 6 Vaccariello, Liz, Editor-In-Chief. Prevention. 2009. Binge-Proof your diet: 6 Foods that keep you full and satisfied. **shine.yahoo.com/event/twoweekturnaround/binge-proof-your-diet-6-foods-that-keep-you-full-and-satisfied-481183/** 7 Sole-Smith, Virginia. 2008. Weight Loss By Design. reFresh/reCharge/reNew, Fall 2008. (Woman's Health Magazine 2007)

Chapter 20: Stress
1 Spears, Britney. 1999.
people.com/people/britney_spears
2 Nachatelo, Melissa. 2003. How to Laugh Off Stress. Natural Health Magazine, March.
3 Eat This Not That. 2009. Men's Health Magazine.
eatthis.menshealth.com/slideshow/30-healthy-foods-arent?cm_mmc=ETNTSNL-_-2009_09_09-_-HTML-body2
4 Henderson, Mark. 2008. Ghrelin stress hormone linked to comfort eating, say Texas researchers. The Times.
timesonline.co.uk/tol/life_and_style/health/article4152037.ece?print=yea&randnum=1252529730881
5 Beattie, Melody. 1948- .
thinkexist.com/quotation/gratitude_unlocks_the_fullness_of_life-it_turns/294749.html
6 cdc.gov/chronicdisease/overview/index.htm
7content.healthaffairs.org/cgi/content/short/hlthaff.28.5.w822
8 Pollan, Michael. September 2009. Big Food vs. Big Insurance. The New York Times.
nytimes.com/2009/09/10/opinion/10pollan.html?scp=4&sq=Michael%20Pollan&st=cse
9 The Worlds Healthiest Foods.
whfoods.com/genpage.php?tname=foodspice&dbid=43
10 Gentry, Reverend Laura. 2009. http://laughinglaura.com
11 Guillemets, Teri. quotegarden.com/stress.html

Chapter 21: Bondage
1 Jameson, Mrs. Anna Brown. 1794-1860.
giga-usa.com/quotes/authors/anna_jameson_a001.htm
2 The Oxford Desk Dictionary and Thesaurus, 2nd Edition. 2001. New York: Berkley Books. Penguin Putnam, Inc.
3 Gittleman, M.S., C.N.S, Ann Louise. 2002. The Fat Flush Plan. McGraw-Hill.
4 Kausman, Rick, Dr. 2001. Calm Eating. Australia: Allen and Unwin.
5 The diet business: Banking on failure. (BBC News World Edition, Feb 5 2003).
news.bbc.co.uk/2/hi/business/2725943.stm

6 Jean Kilbourne, Deadly Persuasion: Why Women and Girls Must Fight the Addictive Power of Advertising (New York: The Free Press, 1999), 27, 58.

Chapter 22: Hedonism and Sensuality
1 Hoffman, Jascha. 2008. Art Teams With Science to Explain It all to You. The New York Times, November 1
2 Robinsin, Maria. 1758-1800.
finestquotes.com/author_quotes-author-Maria%20Robinson-page-0.htm
3 Hirsch, Alan, M.D., F.A.C.P. 1998. Scentsational SEX. Massachusetts: Element Books, Inc.
4 ibid
5 ibid

Chapter 23: Satisfaction
1 Cook, John. The Book of Positive Quotations. 1996. Minneapolis: Fairview Press
2 Gawain, Shakti. 1948- .
en.thinkexist.com/quotation/when_we_create_something-we_always_create_it/327629.html
3 Maltz, Maxwell. 1899-1975.
thinkexist.com/quotation/we_are_built_to_conquer_environment-solve/325454.html
4 Marley, Bob. 1945-1981.
http://www.finestquotes.com/select_quote-category-Satisfaction-page-0.htm
5 Mandino, Og. 1923-1996. http://www.iwise.com/wYqyz
6 Rohn, Jim. 1930-2009.
thinkexist.com/quotation/we_need_a_variety_of_input_and_influence_and/334004.html
7 Rahner, Karl. 1904-1984.
brainyquote.com/quotes/authors/k/karl_rahner.html
8 Frank, Ann. 1929-1945
brainyquote.com/quotes/quotes/a/annefrank110065.html
9 Waitley, Dennis. 1933- .
brainyquote.com/quotes/quotes/d/deniswaitl146
10 Journal of the American College of Nutrition, Vol.20, no.4.
jacn.org/cgi/content/full/20/4/327

11 Esquire Magazine. May 2006.

Chapter 24: Fashion and Media
1 Lauren, Ralph. 1939- .
thinkexist.com/quotation/i_don-t_design_clothes-i_design_dreams/223088.html
2 Karan, Donna. In Style: 2007 Instant Style. January 17.
splendicity.com/articles/todays-fashion-quote-by-donna-karan-101/
3 Thomas, Pauline Weston. Fashion-Era.com
fashion-era.com/bras_and_girdles.htm#The%20Symington%20Side%20Lacer
4 Wilde, Oscar. 1854-1900.
best-quotes-poems.com/fashion-quotes.html
5 de Givenchy, Hubert. 1927- .
educators.fidm.edu/educators/classroom-reso- urces/fashion-qoutes.html
6 Armani, Georgio. 1934- . http://modelbehavior.tumblr.com/
7 Winfrey, Oprah. 2008. What I Know For Sure. O, The Oprah Magazine, June
8 Peat, Ray. Psychological research in the U.S.S.R., 1966. Concerning the Decisive Role of Afferent Systems in Nervous Activity. raypeat.com/articles/
9 Lauren Ralph. 1939- .
evancarmichael.com/Famous-Entrepreneurs/1895/Ralph-Lauren-Quotes.html
10 Crisp, Quentin. 1908-1999.
brainyquote.com/quotes/quotes/q/quentincri104601.html
11. Dyer, Wayne. 1940- .
thinkexist.com/quotation/begin_to_see_yourself_as_a_soul_with_a_body/203856.html
12 The New Oxford American Dictionary (NOAD). 2nd Edition. 2005. Oxford University Press.
oxfordamericandictionary.com/

Other sources:
momswhothink.com/diet-and-nutrition/height-weight-chart.html

wikipedia.org/wiki/Jean_Nidetch
en.wikipedia.org/wiki/Twiggy

Chapter 25: The Lucky Ones
1 Kennedy, John F. 1917-1963.
betterworld.net/quotes/endhunger-quotes-3.htm
2 Buck, Pearl S. 1892-1973.
cultureofpeace.com/quotes/endhunger-quotes.htm
3 Brockovich, Erin. 1960- .
cultureofpeace.com/quotes/endhunger-quotes.htm
4 Williamson, Marianne. 1952- .
thinkexist.com/quotation/personal_transformation_can_and
_does_have_global/330216.html
5 Bridges, Jeff. 1949- .
cultureofpeace.com/quotes/endhunger-quotes.htm
6 Lorca, Federico Garcia. 1898-1936.
hondurasnews.com/2009/08/31/chief-justice-sierra-resigns/
7 Kristof, Nicholas D. 2010. World's Healthiest Food. The New
York Times, January 3, 2010

Chapter 26: Beauty and Balance
1 anon.
thinkexist.com/quotation/every_time_you_see_a_beautiful_
woman-just/184664.html
2 Christy Turlington: Beauty and Balance. June 2001.
Psychology Today psychologytoday.com/print/24105?page=2
3 Turlington, Christy. 1960- .
brainyquote.com/quotes/authors/c/christy_turlington_2.html
4 Roosevelt, Franklin D. 1882-1945.
brainyquote.com/quotes/quotes/f/franklind119525.html
5 Gibran, Kahlil. 1926. The Prophet 19th printing 1976. Borzoi
Book, Alfred A Knopf, Inc.
6 Bacon, Sir Frances. 1561-1626.
brainyquote.com/quotes/quotes/f/francisbac117825.html
7 ideafinder.com/history/inventions/potatochips.htm
8 MacPherson, Elle. 1964 - .
brainyquote.com/quotes/quotes/e/ellemacphe330379.html

Chapter 27: Comfort Food for Chefs
1 Hopkins, Kate. 2005. Accidental Hedonist. **accidentalhedonist.com/index.php?title=what_is_comfort_fo od&more=1&c=1&tb=1&pb=1**
2 Child, Julia. 1912-2004. **famousquotes.psyphil.com/julia-child/quote/41153/**

Index

Notes

Am I Really Hungry?

Am I Really Hungry?

Notes

Am I Really Hungry?